FROM THE UNIVERSE WITH LOVE

You're Guide to Understanding Synchronicities, Signs, and Spiritual Awakenings to Find Harmony, Happiness, Healing, and Purpose in Your Life.

Belle Motley

© **Copyright 2021 - All rights reserved.**

The content contained within this book may not be reproduced, duplicated or transmitted without direct written permission from the author or the publisher.

Under no circumstances will any blame or legal responsibility be held against the publisher, or author, for any damages, reparation, or monetary loss due to the information contained within this book, either directly or indirectly.

Legal Notice:

This book is copyright protected. It is only for personal use. You cannot amend, distribute, sell, use, quote or paraphrase any part, or the content within this book, without the consent of the author or publisher.

Disclaimer Notice:

Please note the information contained within this document is for educational and entertainment purposes only. All effort has been executed to present accurate, up to date, reliable, complete information. No warranties of any kind are declared or implied. Readers acknowledge that the author is not engaged in the rendering of legal, financial, medical or professional advice. The content within this book has been derived from various sources. Please consult a licensed professional before attempting any techniques outlined in this book.

By reading this document, the reader agrees that under no circumstances is the author responsible for any losses, direct or indirect, that are incurred as a result of the use of the information contained within this document, including, but not limited to, errors, omissions, or inaccuracies.

Contents

Introduction 1

The Awakening 5

Vibration 13

Signs and Synchronicities 23

Signposts; Understanding What I See 31

Intuition, Consciousness, and the Subconsciousness 41

Purpose 53

Letting Go 73

Conclusion 83

References 87

A Free Gift for You!

In the **"Vibe Guide,"** you will learn...

- 15 techniques to raise your vibrations and stay in a high frequency

- How to manifest your desires

- How to find peace...

and so much more!

Go to bellemotley.com to receive your free gift!

www.bellemotley.com

Introduction

Spiritual Awakening! What is it exactly? It is something that comes from inside you. The initial manifestations of awakening can be a cause of anxiety and disorientation. The way a person perceives life is about to undergo a major change. The awakening is the first symptom. The problem is identifying it and working with it so that a new wholeness of life slowly unfolds. This changed vision is definitely desirable, as people who have gone through it know. A much more complete vision of life is a path to happiness and contentment.

Today, humans are in the midst of a crisis of identity and social unrest. This may not be apparent, but if one looks closely, it is there. Men and women are fixed upon an unending race towards some goal, wealth, success, or fame. This headlong plunge into life is often the cause of mental distress which envelopes so many people. Anxiety, depression, and a social disconnect tend to be the results. A sense of always being on edge is the emotion that most people feel today, along with a continuous feeling of not attaining the desired goal. This frustration affects people's lives in different ways, some *severe.*

However, a feeling of dissatisfaction may not always be a bad thing. It could be an inner voice trying to communicate something - something important. It is this voice that needs attention.

If this feeling has begun to affect your life and interpersonal skills, the matter needs to be resolved. This book is about such a voyage of discovery! It will tell you the symptoms that indicate a spiritual awakening against stress about a particular problem or incident. If the latter, it will pass away by itself. If the former, then it is here to stay, and you must address it. However, the great thing about this is that it is a gift that could change your life forever!

The author, Belle Motley, is someone who has been through all the trials and tribulations of spiritual awakening and has the knowledge and vision to act as a guide; She had created a great life but quickly lost everything. This resulted from losing her faith and trust in the Divine that all would be well. Life got hard; she couldn't handle it and didn't have the tools that today are so readily available. This led to active addiction. It was a downward spiral until it was nearly the end of her; there was little hope she would survive. She was fortunate enough to find recovery, which got her back on track and onto the path to spiritual awakening, steadily putting her life back together. Today, she is a spiritual guide and lightworker. Her personal experience with the ups and downs of life is significant. **It is often at our darkest hour that we find the brightest light.**

Let's see what this book contains and what it can do for you.

First, it will give you the power to understand your symptoms of unrest. That is *always* the first step: understanding what is eating away from the inside. Without this recognition, nothing much can happen. That is the first tenet of spirituality - *to know*!

Next, you will understand how to deal with the symptoms that have begun to manifest themselves. And deal with those around you who are mystified at your sudden change of attitude. Not everyone is going through a spiritual awakening simultaneously, which may cause some unrest. The chances are that not a single individual around you is going through this process. This is why you may hear, "What's wrong with you?" or "You never behaved in this manner; what's gotten into you?" If someone is also undergoing an awakening, that person will immediately empathize with you. It takes one to know one!

Slowly, the book will take you through several crucial topics, which are of great importance once the journey has begun. Like in any discipline, spirituality, too, has its steps. Awakening of the inner self is just the beginning. It's how you handle yourself that is critically important. Several obstacles will arise, which must be dealt with, and the author will provide you with the steps required to deal with those obstacles, which are, at times, quite formidable. The ego is not likely to take a backseat during the journey. Apart from the ego, family and friends' attempts at dissuading you from doing what you are doing is another obstacle. To them, you are behaving abnormally, even *crazily*! Spiritual journeys are deeply personal, and as you read the book, you will understand why.

The ultimate goal is to be in spiritual harmony with the world around you. No turning back once the path has been chosen. To be solid on the way and confident that the course is correct, certain aspects of reality need to be decoded, and the underlying truth needs to be grasped. This book will show you how.

That sense of despair and unrest that seems to permeate your life is the start of a new journey. You need to see it and act. Prepare yourself with the knowledge and the guidance of someone who has been through the process. This book offers a road map of what to do and how to do it. Answers to all the questions are here. The author will take you through the signposts and their meanings chapter by chapter. Each step needs guidance, which is what this book is for. Some people tend to lose their way and return to their previous approach to life, unaware that a great gift has just passed them by.

Remember: this is a game-changing adventure, such as you have never experienced. So move ahead with courage and determination. You can do it!

Chapter 1
The Awakening

What exactly is a "spiritual awakening"? Today's life is fast-paced; there is very little time to analyze thoughts carefully. There is too much input coming in all at once to give anyone enough time to sort through it. There is also a lot of misinformation out there. To begin with, let us examine 'perception' as a concept.

A change in one's perception about something, in particular, is probably just that. People's perceptions change as they grow older or are privy to new facts. Advertising may change perception subtly about some specific product or lifestyle. These changes are normal ones that affect everyone differently. They happen at a basic level and do not affect life profoundly. Most people are not even aware of these altered perceptions. They are treated as decisions, the freedom to choose. This is not to say that a significant change in perception couldn't lead to an awakening!

Another change that happens to people frequently is acquiring new insight into a particular issue. Now, this can be almost anything: an insight into a work process that makes it better or a relationship. These are changes that affect the person, but they are not spiritual changes by any means. They are reactions to external stimuli and do not arise from within the self. So now, onto the real spiritual awakening - what it is.

Spiritual awakening is something that starts from within oneself. It is ultimately an internal flowering. In the beginning, of course, it may cause a complete feeling of disorientation. This is because the entire world has been turned upside down. However, once you deal with it, a completely new and glorious view of the connectedness of all things takes shape. A new feeling of wholeness will be the gift of this transformative experience.

However, not all spiritual awakenings work the same way. Some are gradual and subtle, with slight hints that try to steer you into another lane. A feeling of disconnect with the material aspect of life is one powerful sign. When things like cars, houses, furniture, and all the other items of modern life begin to lose their importance, a spiritual awakening is happening. This lack of desire and attachment to objects is integral to any spiritual journey. It means that the power of the ego is diminishing in its ability to control your mind and body. The ego gives desire, and it is the ego that makes a person define him or herself.

Letting go of external objects is a definite indication that something different is trying to surface. Worried that you are turning into some sort of hermit? Don't be! It's just a new awareness of reality.

Manifestations of Awakening.

Spiritual awakening may show up in any of the following ways:

- A feeling of dissatisfaction with life.
- A sudden sense of heightened conviction.
- A deep sense of calm and peace.
- A sense of being connected with the environment.
- A feeling of increased happiness and bliss.
- A sense of loneliness and disconnect.
- A hint of a second sight, also known as 'intuition.'

Now, let's try to understand the signs of a spiritual awakening in a little more detail. The feeling that one's life is not going in the right direction is an indicator. A sense of unfulfillment slowly takes hold. The appearance of this feeling is gradually applying the brakes on daily activities and causing a person to undergo introspection. What's the point in carrying on if it does not satisfy? Why am I attached to these things?

This introspection is the first step. The inner voice is trying to help you get rid of illusions that beset most people's lives. It is essentially the questioning of why certain things are important. Suddenly, realization dawns that what one thinks is real and desirable is just an illusion. These are just projections of the mind, not the actual reality. This sort of awakening can happen suddenly or develop over a period of time. However, it usually begins to affect the mind when it is consistently present and refuses to go away. The trick is to sit down and analyze your thoughts. Why are things not satisfying? Is it because you feel that you are doing something wrong? Or is it something else? A little due diligence will slowly reveal the truth. Serious and unbiased thinking, please!

When a feeling of unusual energy fills the body, it signifies spiritual awakening. Everything seems brighter than before, and sometimes everything seems bathed in luminescence. This energy is there in the external world, but you cannot see it until the spirit enhances vision. Remember that this spirit is inside everyone; it's just lying low. The ego is the dominant factor, the force which usually controls the mind and activities of everyone. When the soul or spirit - call it what you will - springs to life and begins to act, a spiritual awakening occurs. This new vision of reality is exhilarating. Everything looks brighter! Flowers look more colorful and seem to be glowing with some form of inherent energy! The whole world is alight. It's a great feeling, and the person wonders why they did not see it before. This, then, is reality. As you stare in wonder at this newfound beauty of all things, your mind will slowly expand to fit this new vision into it. It is necessary to be aware of it and to want it sincerely. You may not have noticed yet, but it has lit up your soul, as well! A message from the author, "when my journey first began, I was walking down the street, beaming with joy and repeatedly saying thank you in my mind. Out of nowhere, two small birds began chasing each other and flying around my legs; I felt like Cinderella! Gratitude is such an important part of spirituality. When you are thankful, you are telling the Universe, more of this, please! You will naturally manifest more wonderful things in your life."

A deep sense of peace and calm sometimes invades the mind. A feeling of desire to slow down typically comes with it. This sensation is the first glimmer of reality, the fact that the importance of all external factors is just illusory. Likewise is the pace to keep up with these external forces. As you step back and look closely, the desire to hold onto things diminishes. Once these external factors lose their importance, a sense of peace and calm descends, the comparison of which can be something like suddenly getting off the merry-go-round: the world of illusion was taking you round and round! And to keep up with this illusory world, continuous involvement in thought and action was the real cause of anxiety, stress, and unhappiness. The inner spirit has just revealed the truth. Consider yourself blessed!

The sudden feeling that all Nature is connected to you is a spiritual revelation. In reality, everything is connected, but we don't see it because of our partitioned worldview. The movie 'Avatar,' directed by James Cameron, used this astral connection. All ancient civilizations were aware of this and respected it. To them, Earth was always Mother Earth. The Native Americans did not want to dig into the Earth for minerals or coal. They said it was sacrilege to dig into the Great Mother to get at her bones. It is a great realization, one which needs to be nurtured. Feeling this oneness brings serenity and a greater sense of peace and belonging, where a web connects every tree, plant, bird, or animal, the web of life. In some ancient cultures, every person was meant to have a spirit soul. It could be a particular tree or some specific animal. The belief was that any harm done to that particular tree or animal was identical to harm being done to the person. A feeling of identity with Nature will perhaps save our environment one day. Also, here is an interesting thing: if you allow Nature to speak to you, it *will*. All the great painters of Nature knew this secret. So the next time you see someone talking to a tree, go up to him and pat him on the back. He's a kindred soul! They also love hugs, as we do!

An exalted feeling of happiness could signify that something spiritual is slowly manifesting. The ordinary sense of joy is a transient one - it lasts for only so long. The feeling of happiness resulting from acquiring something, like a new car, house, dress, and so on, is transitory. It slowly disappears after a while, and something new is required to bring it back. Yet, when a spiritual awakening creates a sense of happiness, that remains because it is not based on external elements but comes from within the self. It is the soul creating this joy as a first step towards understanding the true nature of life. If this feeling is analyzed carefully, no apparent reason can be found. It is the spirit awakening. Enjoy it, and try to hang on to it, because it is true happiness, the real thing!

Is a feeling of loneliness creeping up on you? Are you better off in solitude? If so, these symptoms need to be examined carefully. They are probably a message from inside you, telling you to disengage from the hurly-burly of modern life. However, at the outset, please be aware that if the symptoms intensify and a form of depression begins to take hold, consult a medical professional.

It is necessary to sift through the feeling. The desire for solitude can be a spiritual need. Check to see if you are happy when you are by yourself. If that is the case, then it is a spiritual awakening. The desire to just stand away from crowds and noise is generally a sign that another aspect of your mind is trying to say something. When the spirit begins to unfold itself, it wants introspection. The reason is easy to understand. The spirit is inside you; therefore, one needs to turn inwards to listen to its voice. To do this means moving away from the external disturbances a little. The inner voice, to be heard, needs silence. The din of the external world makes it inaudible, which explains the need for solitude. Anyone who treks through the mountains or forests knows the power of this silence. It is the strange power of being alone - solitude. It may lead to a disconnect with society in general, but that's nothing to worry about, rest assured. It's a temporary phenomenon, and when the voice has had its say, you will re-enter society feeling a lot better and with newfound wisdom, which will surprise others.

Intuition is a faculty of which everyone has heard. Everyone has it, but for some, it is stronger than others. It is like a muscle and needs to be used. Typically, some people say, when an intuitive feeling turns out to be correct, it's merely a coincidence. However, as the seers have always maintained, nothing in this world is a 'coincidence.' Everything has a purpose. A spiritual awakening heightens this faculty. It is like a sense that can foresee events. Normal intuition is infrequent and not always felt. A heightened sense, on the other hand, is present almost always. It is a sense which forewarns when danger is imminent and works to show you the way. It helps you navigate your way through life, acting as an invisible guide, as a spirit guide; in fact, it is a spirit guide or guardian angel! Your personal spirit guide, the presence of this power helps connect you spiritually with other like-minded people. You will intuitively know when you meet another spiritually awakened person.

Now that you know some of the signs that could indicate a spiritual awakening is happening, a few points must be kept in mind.

To start with, please understand that spiritual awakenings don't follow a timetable or even a set sequence of events. They can emerge and flow in their own way. This is different for each individual. Depending on the power of the awakening, the effects might be subtle or forceful. For example, the initial awakening might begin straightaway with a sudden sense of loneliness coupled with a feeling of disconnect. These two things may appear together. It is necessary to understand this and deal with it. How do you deal with it?

The best way is to sit quietly and ponder or meditate on the new elements in your thoughts. Why do you feel lonely? Where did this feeling come from, and why has it appeared in your life? Let's try and get at the reasons.

It is known that spiritual awakening comes to a person when they are ready for it. That is to say, their soul, on its numerous journeys, has reached a point where the Divine presence needs to make its identity known. Making itself known requires the person to look inside and contemplate this in silence; hence, loneliness. In order to attain this silence, it is necessary to cut off ties with the external world of impressions. The voice which is getting ready to speak needs this utter and complete silence and inward-turning attention. That's why loneliness is a symptom of a spiritual awakening.

The point is that loneliness might be accompanied by a feeling of disenchantment with everyday life. The two feelings together can throw anyone off balance. It is a difficult situation to handle. Once again, the trick is to analyze the feelings and try to make sense of them. Not easy, I grant you, but if you stick to it, you will certainly see the light. How much time does this take? It could be days, weeks, or even longer. It would greatly help if you could find a spirit guide, maybe someone you know or read about, who is accessible. A group that you can join is also beneficial. However, you can do this by yourself.

Meditation is a great way to handle this. Sit quietly in a place where you feel comfortable and are not likely to be disturbed. Sit silently, close your eyes, and let your thoughts go. Keep your spine straight for good energy flow. The first thing you notice will be that random thoughts or visions will race through your mind. Don't worry; let that happen. Over time, you will see that these images are slowing down, and the mind is beginning to settle. It is then that the inner voice will appear. Be assured that you will be able to identify it. It's like nothing else you have ever heard before. It isn't usually some voice *actually speaking*; it's more often a sudden sense of realization - the light shines, and everything becomes clear! It is a blessed vision mentioned by all those who have seen it!

There is something to understand about life in general. Everyone is caught up in a rat race; well, almost everyone. The result of this is that our soul light is invisible to us. It is covered by a carnal mesh of layers, effectively blocking its pure light. The mind is entangled in external objects and is prevented from looking inward. It is essential to keep this concept in mind; this is why, when the soul awakens, it tends to draw the person away from external stimuli. To introspect, to peel off the layers of obstruction, is so that the pure light may shine through. That is why loneliness, a feeling of disconnect, occurs.

It is unnerving when it appears; this feeling of disconnect and a sense of dissatisfaction typically accompanies it; a feeling that life, such as it is, does not seem to have any purpose. Be aware that the spirit inside you is trying to turn your thoughts inward. There is nothing to be afraid of; your life is not falling apart. It is just coming to grips with something Divine.

There are many ways in which the basic awakening symptoms mentioned earlier may vary. There are no straight lines in this experience. Each person must tackle it in their own way. Using the guidelines in this book will undoubtedly be of help.

There is, of course, the problem that people around you, family and friends, may not understand what is happening to you. This is normal, so don't sweat it. Not everyone awakes. The reactions you face may be upsetting because you cannot express what you are feeling. They cannot see any reason for your sudden, abnormal behavior (remember, abnormal in their view), and you cannot explain it, either. Just smile and move forward; you have an important journey to make. There is no need to explain yourself; this is your journey. Connect with other like-minded people; you are definitely not alone!

Since some form of solitude and introspection are required to come to terms with what you are experiencing, meditation is the best way. **Meditation, the act of quiet thinking.** No goals need to be set, but several necessary conditions must be adhered to:

- A quiet place - could be a room or an area in the garden.
- It is recommended to sit with your spine straight if you can, but that is not to say you can't meditate lying down.
- Must be free of external noise, aside from maybe some soft music.
- It must be a place that people cannot access easily.
- The cell phone must be switched off - not silent but switched off.

Once such a place is identified, make yourself comfortable. Sit in any convenient position. Then, close your eyes. The whizzing images that you see are a part of your current state of being. They will slow down after a few days. Your mind will calm down. As it does, you will feel something happening. You are now hearing another song, the music of the Universe. Your body is now vibrating at another level. It is in sync with an entirely different stratum, something you didn't know existed. Isn't that great? Slowly, the sensation will pass through your entire body, and a feeling of aliveness will start to take over. You are now tuned in to a higher vibration.

Now, there is one element that you must know and remember. Sometimes, after the initial desire for solitude and meditation, certain **dark thoughts may begin to surface and pass through your mind.** These dark thoughts, which could be about past unpleasant events, are thrown up by the subconscious and need to be addressed. They may last for weeks and make you feel that everything is not going the right way, but it is part of the process of cleansing. Your subconscious needs to be purged. So, allow them passage through your mind. Once they have exhausted themselves, and you have come to terms with them, they will disappear. It is necessary to understand this and not be afraid. Nothing is going wrong; in fact, you are on the right path. These dark thoughts have been there all the time. **In essence, what is happening is the removal of our darkest fears, those that we have suppressed.** These fears have slowly sunk into the subconscious and have affected your life without you being aware of it.

Once sanctified, your inner self will be cleaner and healthier. That's what you need for the path ahead. So do not be afraid; face them with courage, and they will soon leave you in peace. *It is also known as the "Dark Night of the Soul."* This means that the past journey of the soul, which was colored by material desires, anger, and jealousies - among other thoughts and actions, is now appearing. So do not worry, and most of all, do not be afraid. This is part of the journey you are about to make, and it is going to be amazing!

Chapter 2
Vibration

Let us see what vibrations really mean. It is now a scientific fact that everything is composed of atoms, neutrons, protons, and many smaller particles, molecules, or entities. These are constantly in motion. With everything whizzing around, these tiny particles produce a form of vibration. These vibrations, in their turn, are affected by the nervous system. The neural networks in the brain are constantly sending out signals to various parts of the mind, heart, and body. The heart and other organs respond to these signals. For example, when faced with danger, the brain releases adrenaline. This heightens our response to fear and prepares the body for flight. It is known as the "fight or flight" hormone. Similarly, there are pleasure hormones, which cause delight and joy. These, too, are released by our brain.

These pleasure hormones are typically released when we do something we consider enjoyable, like buying new clothes, a new car, or a house. They respond to external stimuli. What we are talking about does not rely on external stimuli.

Initially, raising one's vibrations must be a conscious effort. You have to work at it consciously. A low-level vibration means that there is unhappiness, despair, or some other negative issue. As the vibration rises, the mood changes to happiness and bliss. The higher they connect, the better you feel - that's the secret.

Let's see how you can raise your vibration. The first thing is to keep thinking of happy things: events or experiences which make you feel better. Thinking of sad things makes the vibration connect to lower levels, which means your body feels heavier. If you keep a careful watch, you will see that your body feels lighter when truly happy. When a bout of sadness or unpleasantness strikes, the body seems heavy, and the response to anything becomes slow. The trick, then, is to raise your vibration. Positive thoughts do just that! Keeping your mind positive is not easy, but with a bit of effort, it can be done. Make a vow as soon you get up in the morning - only positive thoughts! Banish all negative ones. Think about something you have gratitude towards! As you will see, it isn't a walk in the park at first, but slowly, the habit begins to take hold. You will become aware of your thoughts and be able to stop the negative ones. Try replacing one negative thought with three positive ones. An immediate improvement in your daily life will show up. People will respond to you better, your mood will affect the way you work, and best of all, you are on top of the world. That's a great place in which to be!

Another way of raising your vibration is to use meditation. Here the path is to meditate on the good things in life. Some unhappy and dark thoughts will likely surface but carry on regardless. Let the unpleasant thoughts play themselves out. They need to be sorted and resolved. Continue to focus on the brighter moments. Remember that the more pleasant memories you can focus on, the happier you will be. Happiness helps connect to higher vibrations.

Then, there is the way of bonding with nature. For instance, go for a walk in the park, especially when it is not crowded. When too many people are present is not an ideal atmosphere. You are trying to reach out to nature and connect. This strategy also helps in getting rid of the stress in your mind, which gives rise to negative thoughts and feelings. You really don't need those! Just sit quietly on a park bench. Look around you, stare at the trees and flowers, and let your mind go. It will wander around and come back refreshed. How will you know that you just did something successfully? Examine yourself. Do you feel happier, more peaceful? And your body – does it feel less heavy, like maybe you lost a few pounds of weight? If yes, then your attempt has been a success.

Now it is necessary to go a little deeper into vibration and "connect to Source Energy" - God, the Universe, Higher Power, whatever suits you. Know, without any doubt, that you are an extension of Source Energy; that is, a part of it. You are connected to the Source Energy; only you may not realize it. Once you can keep this important fact in your mind and sincerely believe in it, you will see it. That's the way of awakening.

This connection, which you will slowly come to know, will illuminate ordinary objects and your mind to such an extent that the world becomes completely different. Even your thoughts will begin to reflect this new reality. Everyday objects will glow with an inner light, which they possess, but you have been unable to see because you were tuned in to a lower vibrational level or frequency.

How do you know that you are vibrating at a higher level and are tuned into the Universe? There are several signs which will help you to know.

The first thing is to be mindful. This means being acutely aware of your surroundings and everything you are doing. It isn't just 'knowing'; it is being aware. There is a difference. In the Japanese philosophy called 'Bushido,' this is the most essential step. This awareness will alert you to signals and messages from the spirit world. You certainly don't want to miss those!

Once you are aware of your life, you may find that certain things are repeatedly happening. For example, you may hear the same phrase over and over again. Now that you are aware try and examine why that phrase has come into your life. It is probably trying to tell you something. There are other similar repetitive incidents that you will notice happening. Each of these needs to be examined. For example, a bird may suddenly appear and sit on your window. Why did it come? If it regularly comes, time to pay attention. There are many examples of these indications. It is up to you to spot them.

Now, onto the mystery of numbers. Numbers are very potent symbols, indicating many different things. There is an entire science of numbers and is generally called 'Numerology.' This science tells us that numbers, from 0 to 9, are ruled by various planets. For example, the number '4' is said to be ruled by Uranus; the number '8' by Saturn. Then there is the number '9'. Any number multiplied by nine results in 9. Here's an example: 12x9= 108. Now, add the digits together: 1+0+8=9. Try that with any number, and the result will be the same. Nine is the triplicity of the number '3', the magic number of all ancient mystical systems. A more detailed exposition of numbers is mentioned in a later chapter.

Therefore, number symbols which appear consistently in your life are important. It is certain that if you examine your own life, you will find the predominance of a certain number. This is typically related to your life path number. You will notice that this number will be significant in your life. For example, it may be your marriage date, when you had your first child, the month you were born, or when you got your first job. To find your life path number, do this: write down your date of birth (Ex: 12.5.1982), and then add the digits of the day (1+2=3), and then add that to the month (3+5=8). After that, add the digits of the year (1+9+8+2=20), make a single number by adding (2+0=2). So now we have the following: 8 + 2=10. Now reduce this to a single digit (1+0=1). This number is your life path number and will reappear many times in your life. Important events will be linked to this number, sometimes to multiples of it.

So now you know that numbers play a key part in your life. Look out for them. Certain numbers reappearing in your life means that specific planetary and spiritual influences are operating. If the effects are benign, then that is good for you, but should they be adverse, then it's time to take corrective action. This is one of the benefits of being aware, of being connected. The Universe is sending you a heads-up. Nothing to be worried about; just be aware. That way, you can avoid any harmful influences that may affect your life - more on numbers to come.

Now, we need to talk about intuition. You think of someone, and that person either calls you on the phone or arrives at your doorstep. That isn't a coincidence. That indication came from your connection to spirit. There are numerous ways that you can get a glimpse of the future. These are called "intuitive feelings." An enhanced awareness leads to this faculty becoming more and more active. Most people have had an intuitive flash at some point in their lives. It is a faculty that is dormant in many people. A heightened sense of connection with the spirit world increases this sense immensely. This intuitive faculty may sometimes make you feel that something good is about to happen. It may also warn you about something negative, giving you time to take evasive action, a form of protection, if you examine it carefully. You are not alone and are being Divinely guided. That's a great feeling! When your vibrations are high, that connection is stronger. There are several documented cases where the power of intuition has saved someone's life. There is a link between intuition and the subconscious mind. A detailed write-up is in an upcoming chapter.

Dreams are perhaps the clue to many things; some hidden, some just below the conscious mind. Dreams have been studied by almost all ancient cultures and have been considered extremely important symbols of the cosmos. Dreams can sometimes reveal a deep-seated need you might have but were never aware of. These can sometimes surface to remind you of your desires. Yet, dreams can also be prophetic. The dreams which need to be taken seriously are those that reoccur. If you have the same dream repeatedly, it needs to be examined for content. Dreams often are precursors of actual events. A particular dream might warn you about some activity you plan to undertake. It is a good idea to desist from doing that specific thing, whatever it is. When your vibrations are high, some of these dreams are sure to occur. Study what they say, and then decide. Some dreams show happy and positive situations, and you tend to wake up with high spirits. These sorts of dreams indicate that something good is coming your way or that you are doing things right. Once you raise your vibration, dreams will begin to change. Just be aware of how it changes and what it is trying to say. **Dreams arise from the subconscious mind and surface when the conscious mind is at rest. That's why we dream when we sleep.**

We now come to an important point: how do you know you have raised your vibration? There are several signs which will tell you that you are currently vibrating on a higher level.

We have already spoken about intuition, dreaming, and numbers. **However, there are some very manifest symptoms of an enhanced vibration.** The first is the sudden influx of creative ideas. These thoughts seem to arrive out of nowhere, but they can give you excellent suggestions about many things, from family to work to relaxation. They could be about almost anything! These ideas generally come when the mind is not attached to something external is free to roam. It even happens when a person is just a little absent-minded, in fact. Some of the most remarkable scientific ideas came to people when they were not thinking of anything in particular. When your consciousness is raised, these things happen. Therefore, it is vital to let your mind go free for some time. It may bring back some excellent ideas!

Another peculiar faculty that will slowly begin to manifest itself is *the ability to foresee minor events before they happen.* For example, you may feel that your mother needs help, and moments later, she calls to let you know that she does, in fact, need assistance with something. Weird, right?! But once you awaken and your senses become acute, these prophetic visions will soon multiply. They are the guidance provided by Cosmic Power.

Certain images, which we may come across at random, may illuminate a problem we have been grappling with for some time. These images either provide the solution directly or point you towards the correct answer. The more you meditate and let your senses develop, these elements will frequently appear. The idea is to understand these images and their purpose. Your conscious mind, controlled by the ego, may want you to disregard them but stay focussed, and you will learn the secret.

Another aspect that shows you are now vibrating at a higher level - **your presence, as seen by others, has undergone a subtle change, a change for the better.** It is other people who notice the change. You may not know it at first. Suddenly, you find that new and interesting people are coming into your life. Their arrival makes your life happier and better. They may bring opportunities with them. They may even tell you that you seem to be glowing with some kind of inner light. That is perfectly correct – you *are* glowing! This is the new you!

The vital factor is to stay positive at all times. Thinking positively has immediate results. If you keep a positive outlook for most of the day, you will see that you are attracting more good things than when you are in a negative frame of mind. You can test this anytime you wish. **When you remain positive, this means that your conscious mind is changing.** That is very important to remember; positivity attracts positivity. When you are positive in your outlook, more people will try to meet and talk to you. They will also smile and look happy. It's actually what they are absorbing from your energy or aura. In effect, you are projecting positive vibes onto these people. With a negative view, however, the results are just the opposite. People will tend to avoid you, and even if they can't, they will make excuses to leave you quickly. Negative vibes tend to put off people. These positive and negative vibes are very crucial. That is why it is indispensable to keep a positive mindset as much as possible. *To be positive is engaging with the world.*

Modern life is attached to gadgets, which can be addictive. Stuck in this electronic web, people miss out on some of the most essential things in life. They miss out on sunsets, a beautiful sky, or the magical beauty of a flower. You can still use gadgets but restrict their usage as much as possible. Being immersed in a screen is not doing your eyes any good, either. The important thing to remember is this: if you don't look around you, how can you see something magical when it appears? The appearance may be short-lived, as things of this nature usually are, and you have just missed it. These little signs of beauty speak of something greater, something transcendent. It is necessary to see and absorb, to understand. The whole problem is that people are going through their days in a fog. They are following a routine and seem like they are on autopilot. That dumbs down the finer senses. A machine-like approach to life, perhaps unintended, turns people into, well, machines! And machines don't feel - they just work! That is no life for any human being. We did not come here to behave like machines. We have a mind, an intellect, and emotions. It is necessary to pay attention to this fact, and a spiritual awakening will slowly remove these blinders and make people see the world; *really* see it.

"A mechanical life is not worth living" is a phrase often heard. The reason is easy to see. This sort of life takes people away from the world's important things, such as music and the arts, the things that add value to our existence. A superior sense is completely submerged beneath the daily minutiae of work. That is why spiritual awakening is such a wonderful thing. It peels away the layers of ignorance, and the inner light bursts forth in all its glory.

In Buddhism and all Eastern philosophies, this inner light is meditated upon. It is shrouded by layers of what is called the "ego's mindset." Its light is hidden. The idea is to slowly unravel the outer layers created by the ego and reveal the Pure Light within.

However, the first step is to awaken the spirit which resides inside you. Once you take the first step towards that, you will find that, slowly, your perceptions of life will change.

Take a step forward by being generous towards people. Generosity is a powerful tool. The gratitude you will receive from people is a vibration that will positively affect you. Just extend a helping hand and see what happens. Not only will you receive thanks from people, but your entire persona will change to a happier one. Your whole environment will change for the better. Generous people are admired, and others' attitudes towards you will undoubtedly be positive. So why not take this gift? A gift you can share with the world. Sharing your inner light will not only help you, but it will raise the vibration of our planet! We can change the world!

Another available gift: removal of toxins from the body. Reduce or avoid alcohol. That's one of the ways toxins in the body can be lessened, and reducing toxins means cleansing the system inside. A better digestive system means a better nervous system. The liver, kidneys, and stomach all form an integral part of the whole. Therefore, each one affects the other. In Eastern spiritual systems, the initiate is made to ingest a substance that makes him strenuously throw up.

This is the first step: cleansing the body of toxins. After that, the initiation ceremony begins. We're not recommending you make yourself sick; this is an extreme example. The reduction of toxins directly affects health, and you will be able to see that you feel a lot lighter and better. You will sleep more naturally and perform better in any work you undertake. There is, in fact, more energy.

Now we come to food, music, and media. These are important since we are exposed to them almost all the time. There is a continuous flow of sensory data that a person is exposed to nowadays.

Food, as all ancient cultures knew, is extremely important. You've heard the saying that "we are what we eat." Perfectly true. Eat a lot of leafy vegetables, and reduce consumption of meat. Eat nourishing food, and keep a handle on the quantity you eat. Eat foods with a low caloric density. Overeating once in a while is ok, but don't make it a habit. A smaller meal keeps the body lighter and the mind alert. Overeating causes the body to be drowsy, and the brain begins to slow down. Too much of the body's energy is going into digestion.

Music is today used in the treatment of psychiatric patients. It has a profound effect on the mind. It has been proven that classical music makes plants grow better than Rock or Pop music. That is not to say those two genres are 'bad' just that nature reacts to classical music a lot better. Listen to music that has a calming effect. The easiest way is to check which music relaxes you and enhances your mood. Sometimes, of course, music that excites you is just fine, but try to keep that to a minimum.

The same principle applies to movies. Violent movies or those with an overdose of the macabre are not exactly made to calm your nerves. On the contrary, they are made to excite your senses and sometimes depress your mind. This is precisely the opposite of what is required when trying to enhance your vibration. Television is also a medium that is right there in your house. The rule, which applies to movies, also applies to programs on TV. Some programs positively impact the viewer, and there are those designed to cause sadness and anxiety. The problem is that people tend to identify with the characters on the show. That is why watching shows with a positive element is the better option. These will fill you with uplifting thoughts, which by now you are aware, are one of the essential ingredients of a spiritual awakening.

The following important facet is to surround yourself with beauty. Remove all clutter because this tends to slow down the cosmic rays you are trying to absorb. ***Donate all unnecessary things and clean up your home.*** Bring in items that are pleasing to the eye. That does not mean buying expensive objects. Getting some beautiful art pieces to look at or peaceful landscapes may be a good idea. Keep objects in rooms down to the minimum. Less clutter frees what the Chinese call 'chi,' cosmic energy, which is exactly what you are trying to attract. Keep flowers, as they are one of the best mood uplifters ever, but remember to dispose of them away once they are past their bloom. Dead flowers in the room are a no-no! Touching the flowers gently with your fingers is a great way to feel the glory of creation. Do this in your room, or go to a garden area where flowers are abundant. Drink in the beauty, touch and feel, see and smell. There is one thing you will realize: there are many different greens in nature! There are dark greens, light greens, and yellowish greens, to name a few. There are many shades of color in a single flower! Start looking for these shades. They work wonders for the mind as you begin to see the majesty of creation! Your inner vibration begins to rise to meet the challenge.

Another essential area where you can make changes is people. Start with friends and acquaintances. Surround yourself with people who are outgoing and cheerful by nature. Try and avoid those whose presence is always dispiriting. There are people who are often in some sort of trouble, either real or imagined, and they are ready to decant this into your ears. Keep your distance from these people as much as possible. They bring low-level vibrations with them, which can affect you negatively. You may absorb some of those vibrations. You seriously do not need that! However, there are times when you don't have the option to be away from these people. In this case, protect your energy with prayer and meditation. Your guides and angels are readily available to protect and support you. It is important to ask, though, as they respect our free will.

Since it is imperative to keep your mind positive, try not to get irritated or annoyed by how things are happening around you. There may be people yelling and making a fuss about something. Fussing is easy, but doing something isn't. Your positive energy can contribute to helping fix things. So stay positive, and don't get involved in the negative energy of worry and anxiety. If you find that you are reacting, this is an area that needs your attention. You can't always control what is happening around you, but you can control how you respond. You are in control of your thoughts. With meditation and practice, this will become easier.

Now that you are on your way to a spiritual awakening, there are signs which begin to appear. We deal with these in the next chapter.

Chapter 3
Signs and Synchronicities

The word 'coincidence' is one that you will come across frequently from people who are not aware of what you are doing. When you see something and decode the sighting to someone, be prepared for an odd look and the word 'coincidence,' just smile and carry on. **What are some of the signs and symbols that will tell you that you are now on a higher plane of vibration? And why do they manifest?**

The signs and symbols that you will begin to see mean that the spirit world is trying to get in touch with you. A higher vibration does just that. It opens your consciousness to these cosmic events. At first, these signs may feel creepy and weird and create a sense of apprehension. Fear not! They are trying to tell you something.

One of the things you may notice is **the sudden flickering of a light.** You may be sitting, reading, or watching TV when one of the room's lights starts flickering. Electrical fault? Could be. But if that is the only one flickering, then take notice. Have the light checked, by all means. Chances are you will see that there is nothing wrong with it. Then there is the fact that it does not flicker all the time, only once in a while. Also, it's the only light that behaves in this manner. It could be a message from someone who has passed on. As you progress, you will begin to understand. However, be aware that a sudden blowing of a light bulb is not always a sign of a problem with the electrical outlet or lamp, for that matter. Sometimes, there is no explanation, but you need to pay attention when these events happen. Be aware that they will occur when you are around, not otherwise. These things are meant for you and you alone. The spirit world is trying to tell you something. The best way to deal with this is to sit and concentrate and try to find out what the message is. You may ask if someone is trying to contact you from the other side, or you can just wait for some hint or clue as to the reason. Journaling may also help with this matter. The answers will come as you begin to move forward in your spiritual path. Never fear.

The TV is another place where a strange phenomenon may occur. When you are watching a particular channel, the picture on the screen disappears, there is snow, and then a face appears for a split second and disappears. Then, the program you were watching comes back on normally. Fault in the broadcast? Possibly, but it could also be someone trying to send you a message or just saying hello. Someone close, who is no longer with you.

The important thing to realize is that there is another plane of existence. It is well known that this is of the nature of higher consciousness, something you will begin to tap into as your spiritual awakening progresses.

Everyone who has watched ghost stories on TV or at a movie theater or read books about spirits knows that they announce their presence by lowering the room's temperature. A chill begins to permeate the area. This temperature drop is a sure sign that a spirit is in the immediate vicinity. Check to see if a cold breeze has somehow managed to get in. If not, then there is a presence. What it means is for you to find out. There are no set answers to these things. Note from the author, "when I was a newborn child in my crib, my grandmother felt an icy cold rush of wind over her face and *knew* to go to my room. I was blue and had nearly died; she got there just in time to save my life. Coincidence, I think not."

Apart from these, **there are several other indicators that the spirit world is trying to contact you and send you a message.** Perhaps a clock stops the moment you enter a room. If this does happen, note the time carefully. The numbers that indicate the time are important. What this means is detailed in a later chapter. Yet, be sure that this was an event meant for your eyes. Then there are the orbs found in photographs, digital ones nowadays. These strange balls of light aren't a flare, which is a typical photography issue. It is a ball of light inexplicably present in a picture. There is no reason for its presence. If that happens to you, study the photo carefully. Ask yourself if this could be someone trying to send you a message or make you aware of their presence; was there something happening at the time of the photo that needed special attention? You will know why it's there sooner or later because it will probably reappear until you get it.

Some signs have to do with living creatures. Take, for instance, butterflies. This insect has a short life span and is beautiful to see. It wanders around, sipping honey from flowers. Imagine one coming and hanging around

24 | SIGNS AND SYNCHRONICITIES

you for no apparent reason. In some cultures, butterflies indicate that someone will soon be married. But why has it come? Coincidence? That word again! Always keep in mind that nothing in this world is a coincidence. It's just a label that people use to explain something they cannot really understand.

There is a list of animal signs and their meanings in the next chapter, explaining the significance of different animal sightings.

How do you know that these are signs? Once you are aware of yourself and your surroundings, you will slowly become alert to signs you never knew existed before. It isn't that they were not there. You simply did not recognize them. Start paying attention, and you will quickly realize the cosmic signals. You must also be in a state of mind which wants to receive these signs. Receptivity is very important. Keep your mind open, your senses calm, and your vibrations high. You will receive, never doubt that!

The next point to talk about is: can you ask for signs from the Cosmos? And if so, how do you know that they are signs meant for you?

Let's say you have an issue that you want to resolve, but you are unsure how it should be handled. Sit in a meditative position, mull over the problem, and ask for guidance with all your heart. This is the first step. Without connecting to the inner self, you won't get anywhere. Keep your mind focused, and watch for an image or an inspired thought. You may receive hints which you must decode for yourself. This could come as a sense or a vision. You may not get anything, but this doesn't mean you have failed. A solution might just pop into your mind out of nowhere, or it could mean that the hint is outside, in the external world. Keeping a heightened sense of awareness of yourself and your surroundings, step out to do whatever it is you normally do. **Keep an open mind and pay attention to everything that happens around you. Somewhere in that melee of events is the sign.** You need to spot it. If your desire is strong enough, you will undoubtedly see it. The sign could be anything: a tune, or a particular advertising board, or a phrase someone uses. Signs can come from anywhere. Once you recognize it, you will feel a premonition that this sign is what you were seeking. Analyze the sign, and see how it applies to your particular problem. Is there a hint of a solution? If so, go with it. In the initial phases, use signs with care. When they provide the solution you seek, you know that the Universe is answering. You are connected to that consciousness!

At times, the sign is startlingly clear. Go with it without hesitation. However, if you are not sure that the sign was for you, you need to go back to meditating on the problem. This is normal, so never feel that you are not making it. The next time around, the sign may be more explicit. It is a question of connection. This is not a sure thing every time you meditate on some problem. So accept that the Cosmos may respond to your call for help after several attempts or when you are meant to have the answer you seek. This is perfectly normal. Believe and have unwavering faith; your answers will come.

Now, we come to an important concept which needs clarification. The root matter of all spirituality is synchronicity and the difference between the ego and the soul.

Before we go into the differences between the ego and the soul, **we will look at another mysterious factor: synchronicity.** This term was given importance by C. G. Jung, a famous psychologist. He discovered that certain events are inexplicably linked to our personal psyche. To put this simply, a "synchronistic event" means an event that happens when a person is thinking of something, and they see or notice that the event seems to link to their thoughts or feelings. Jung found that this synchronicity was in some way connected to the space-time continuum. While that is probably true, what is a fact is that these things happen to people. The trick is to perceive these as messages from the spirit world, not just chance happenings. Synchronicity is an important aspect of spiritual awakening. The more alert you are, the more these events will make sense. It sounds incredible that external events vibe with our thoughts. But, that they do; is a fact!

Now we will discuss the ego and the soul. There is a difference between the two, and it is a significant difference. The ego is that sense which gives us our persona. It provides us with a feeling of who we are, our importance - most often perceived to the world - and works to interact with the external world. It is mainly rooted in the conscious mind because it deals with our daily actions. Feelings of anger, hurt, fear, and jealousies are some of the functions of the ego. It is who we are. That is why some people use the term 'egotistic' when referring to anyone who is self-centered and selfish. The ego, when unchecked, does make a person behave like that. **The problem is that the ego hinders any kind of spiritual awakening.**

26 | SIGNS AND SYNCHRONICITIES

When people are so full of themselves that they think the world is at their feet, their spiritual path is blocked. For those people, to throw away their sense of self-importance and begin the inward journey will be a great struggle. The ego is a powerful thing and not easily overcome. To get it to come to heel is challenging, to say the least, but it can be done. These people take offense at the slightest hint of their faults. That is the first barrier. That is why it is essential to learn to look inward and not rely on our external facade, the one we present to the world because that is a creation of the ego and is not the true self.

The true self lies within everyone. It is the Soul. This is part of the Great Soul of the Universe. Our partitioned view of the world prevents us from seeing it. The typical vision of people sees everything as separate. That is an illusion. It is veiled by what is called 'Maya.' Every single thing in this world partakes of this one consciousness. Imagine the sea coming into a rocky beach. When low tide occurs, the sea recedes, leaving pools of water behind in the rock crevices. This water will again become part of the sea when the tide next comes in. These small pools are what we are: part of the ocean but perceived as separate pools, an illusion of separation that never really exists. It is essential to understand this fact clearly. It is the very basis of spirituality.

The soul is pure light. It is the Godhead inside everyone. But it is entirely covered by layers of a carnal mesh which prevents us from perceiving it. The poet Browning in his poem 'Paracelsus' puts it beautifully:

> Truth is within ourselves; it takes no rise
> From outward things, whate'er you may believe.
> There is an inmost centre in us all,
> Where truth abides in fullness; and around
> Wall upon Wall, the gross flesh hems it in,
> This perfect, clear perception-which is the truth.
> A baffling and perverting carnal mesh
> Binds it, and makes all error; and to know,
> Rather consists in opening out a way
> Whence the imprisoned splendour may escape,
> Than in effecting entry for a light
> Supposed to be without.

In these lines is the secret of what the soul is. The 'light' the poet talks about is the light of the soul, the Pure Consciousness. The Godhead. That is what the Soul is. This is why an inward meditation is required to see it, to realize it! A spiritual awakening is a way to become aware of the presence of this light. **Once the mind turns inward, the layers begin to fall away, and the Soul's presence is felt.** The important point to note is that the light is not outside you. It resides inside everyone. The whole idea is to get to know it, to let it shine forth in all its transcendent glory! Anybody who has seen this once will never be the same again. Their perspective on life will have changed completely. In this connection, it could be useful to examine near-death experiences. There are thousands of recorded cases. When a person's heart stops, the doctors try to revive the patient. Until the brain has died, death is not diagnosed in modern medicine. Now, patients who suffered from this condition have had what is called an *"out of body experience."* They saw themselves floating above their own body in the operating room and looking down at what the doctors were doing to them. It was like looking at their own deceased bodies. The thing is to understand what they saw at the precise moment that their hearts stopped beating.

Every single person said that they saw a tunnel of light, extremely bright. They began to float through this tunnel. An overwhelming sense of peace pervaded their minds and bodies. It was as if they were in paradise. Then came images of their loved ones, and they returned to their bodies. All of the people who went through this experience felt that their lives had changed irrevocably – they had no fear of death anymore! The reason? They knew that the journey into consciousness was one of peace and happiness. Life had more meaning than ever.

It must, however, be remembered that the ego cannot entirely be removed. Its function is necessary for our daily lives. For example, to interact with people, to work, and so on. However, once the inner voice is heard, it will be like a mentor and guide you in your journey through life. The trick is to keep the ego under control. This is not easy. Our feeling of self-importance and individuality is firmly rooted in our psyche. To tone down these feelings so that the authentic Self can show itself and be heard is a crucial journey, but it takes time and commitment.

It is essentially a rewiring of the neural network in your brain. Habits and feelings tend to connect the neural networks in a certain way. Daily habits, actions, and reactions to events are also wired into that network. To rewire means modifying what we think and how we think. That is why meditation and self-awareness are required to have a spiritual awakening. These systems slowly alter the neural network. It is important here to mention that the brain runs everything, from the movement of our limbs to feelings of happiness and sadness. Hormones secreted by the brain give rise to feelings of pleasure, anger, and depression. It is the most vital of the vital organs. **Perception, too, is controlled by the brain. Meditation alters those perceptions.**

When we go a little deeper into meditation, it is necessary to understand that it essentially targets the pineal gland. This gland plays a critical part in the functioning of the brain. Neuroscientists are still not sure of all its functions. What is known is that it is part of the endocrine system in the brain and that it controls the secretion of a hormone called 'melatonin,' which helps people sleep at night. It is also responsible for the release of other hormones. It is, thus, an important gland. In spiritualism, the pineal gland controls what is known as the "Third Eye" or a powerful sense of intuition. Once this eye is opened, events are known before they happen. The pineal gland is a cone-shaped gland situated in the epithalamus of the brain. It is at the back of the center of your forehead. It is enough to know that it is the gateway to cosmic connection with the transcendent consciousness.

Remember that the meditation you are practicing has an effect on this very important of glands, but in the beginning, try not to focus on this aspect.

Chapter 4
Signposts; Understanding What I See

The first concept is the matter of free will. Certainly, it appears that people make decisions, and those decisions are theirs and theirs alone. There is no other factor affecting those choices, but if we sift through this concept, we will see that we make decisions based on who we have made ourselves to be. This means that we have come into this world with certain ingrained Karma, which explains who we are. We are here to play out a specific part - like in a play - and we will make suitable decisions to do it. Some may disagree with this concept. The idea of the Soul going through several births is not acceptable to all. No matter. What the skeptics cannot explain, however, is the phenomena of child prodigies, to take just one example. How can a 5-year-old play piano concertos? How can a seven or 8-year-old solve mathematical problems taught at a university level? The only explanation is that they brought those skills from their previous incarnation. There does not seem to be any other explanation.

Therefore, the first thing to believe in is that the Universe - or Cosmic Power - is trying to lead you along the path. It is the path which you should be following. The practitioners of Zen call this "flowing in the current of the Tao." Using the limited amount of free will granted to humans to go against this path means disappointment and trouble.

So, how do we follow the path and use the guidance provided by the Universe? The first thing to do is recognize that there is a benevolent power out there that is looking out for you. Once this is accomplished, the next step is to accept that guidance.

Divine guidance typically comes in the form of dreams, signs, and symbols. Once you are ready to accept guidance, you will recognize these signs. As you progress in your journey, you will slowly learn to work with these signs.

Remember this, though: signs and symbols don't have the same meaning for everyone. They are personal and apply to your state of being only. You may find these lines repetitive, but they are essential. We will now examine some signs which signify various things.

Let's work with a real-life experience.

"One day, I was talking with my now dear friend for the first time on the phone; he suddenly spotted a hawk hovering above and asked whether a hawk meant anything to me. My response was, yes, that is my Spirit Animal! It was a sign from the Universe that we were spiritually connected, and our goals were aligned.

Events such as these occur. They *have* to be recognized.

The sudden appearance of animals, birds, and insects is significant. If they appear while you have been pondering a situation or looking for an answer, think about what it could mean for you at that time. If any of the following animals become your Spirit Guide, or you wish to invoke them as your Spirit Guides, then the qualities associated with each are either part of you or something you need to acquire. Remember, though, that you may see these animals or birds in your dreams and not necessarily physically.

Bear: Strength and courage are of the essence. Bears are animals who are known to be extremely strong. Therefore, the sighting of a bear may be telling you to strengthen your inner resources and face the world from a position of courage. It is a sure indication that you need to change your stance to include the sense of readiness to take on anything.

Badger: Patience and resourcefulness and the ability to survive in difficult circumstances. This animal is a benign creature known for its ability to persevere and build its homes. They are gentle creatures, and if you dream about them, it is a sign telling you to persevere in whatever you are doing, but gentle perseverance.

Blue Jay: This bird is a very spirited one and will fight if threatened. It is clever enough to back down when it feels that it cannot win, though. A blue jay is loud in its call, indicating defiance by its resonant tone. The message, which such a bird brings, is one of being voluble about grievances and not silently absorbing everything. However, it also denotes caution in whatever protests are being made to prevent things from getting worse. Just establish the perimeters of your life so that people know which lines not to cross.

Cardinal: This bright red bird is a treat to witness. The vibrant color immediately uplifts the mind. It is said that in the Christian tradition, they represent the Soul-nature of Man. Since these birds stick to their mates for life, a close look at homelife is indicated. Its cry is cheery and brings with it a feeling of joy. Some say that the nature of cardinals is feminine. This means that the feminine or softer side of the mind needs more attention. There is a feminine side inside a man and a masculine side inside a woman.

Cats: These animals are a part of mysticism. The ancient Egyptians considered them sacred. They are indicators of the power to overcome. Cats move around silently and can be independent. They may disappear for a day or two and then return. This shows that a bit of independent thinking may be in order. However, cats tend to demonstrate that you should rely on your intuition and inner strength more than your physical power.

Crow: Generally, crows are known as carrion eaters, and they are looked upon with disdain. However, crows are survivors as well as brilliant. Almost second to none, the crow has a strong sense of picking up the impending danger. Alertness and the ability to survive against all odds seem to be the message. In addition, the crow has a sharp memory, remembers those who feed it and shies away from those who would do them harm - a very human trait. Therefore, it is saying that you should love those close and stay away from those that would harm you.

Hawk: This bird is known for its incredible vision and the ability to fly high in the sky. It is from these high altitudes that hawks can see their prey. The reference is obviously to a heightened sense of perception and the courage to look at everything from a greater perspective. In spirituality, that is precisely the goal: to rise above the mundane.

Hummingbird: This bird is one of God's incredible creations. It is one of the smallest birds out there. Its colors are beautiful, it has the ability to hover (think helicopters), and its long beak can delve into any flower to sip nectar. The hummingbird has the additional capability to flit in any direction: forwards, backward, or sideways. The hovering nature of this little bird is an indication to move your mind to a plane from which vantage point you can observe life in its inexplicable complexity. It's akin to reaching the top of a mountain and looking around. This bird is said to have healing powers. Maybe it's time to heal yourself by taking time off and concentrating on more spiritual matters?

Lizard: Seeing or dreaming of lizards means something new might be in the wind. It could be the start of some new project. It is also a sign that energy renewal is required; that means the inner spiritual energy.

Owl: It is a nocturnal bird and is considered a wise one. Owls have always been associated with wisdom. It is a sign that intuition is essential. This creature also indicates that the Spirits' wisdom is necessary as a guide, looking beyond the conscious world.

Pigeon: These gentle and docile birds symbolize peace, but they have an outstanding talent for homing into locations where they have been. In older times, they were used as messengers… and they still are! They bring the most important message of peace and goodwill. Pigeons are also susceptible to atmospheric changes. Therefore, the message is this: stay tuned into your environment and practice peace and goodwill towards all.

Raven: Now, some consider the sighting of a raven to be a bad omen, but omens are subject to different interpretations. Some believe that a raven indicates new beginnings. The best way would be to see what it portends to you. It could be the harbinger of good news.

Robin: The sight of this red-breasted bird indicates hope, that being the eternal hope which springs up in the human mind. It is a sign of renewal and points to the beginning of something new. It has positive messages which indicate that good times are coming.

Seagull: A seagull soars, dives, and sometimes just drifts over land and ocean. The idea which this bird seems to indicate is that of stepping back from the vagaries of life and taking a broader view of it. When viewed from a higher perspective, there are always things that can show a different picture. This elevated view of the composite of life will help resolve and eliminate unnecessary issues cluttering your own.

Snakes: These reptiles are indicative of great wisdom and power. Mystics in every country treat snakes with high regard. They are the repositories of arcane wisdom. If this animal appears in your dreams, be ready to engage with your inner self. Mother Nature requires your attention. It is also the symbol of rejuvenation. Snakes shed their skins and generate a new one - a form of transformation!

Now, we look at some of the insect signs that may signify messages from beyond.

Here is a personal incident from the author's life:

"I was thinking of my mother, who had passed away. I was sitting in my car and about to drive off when a dragonfly flew by. I noticed it especially because she loved dragonflies, and of course, I was thinking of her at that moment. I got the feeling that it was her. She returned and kept buzzing around the car. I sat, watched, and knew that my mother was sending a message. She was saying that she was okay and not to fear; she is always with me."

Ants: These insects are present everywhere. They are patient and diligent creatures. They also have a sense of perseverance, as anybody who has observed them knows. Ants work together in cooperation for the benefit of the colony. So, the indications seem to be diligence, perseverance, and cooperation. Ants are also extremely hardworking. Therefore, hard work, coupled with a lot of patience and perseverance, might be what is signified. In certain cultures, the appearance of ants in the house indicates the arrival of prosperity. Do your own investigation, though. What is it doing for *you*?

Bees: Highly organized and productive creatures, bees collect and store honey for the benefit of all hive members. The sighting of bees is a sign of balance. They fly around, collecting nectar, settle on flowers, and sit while peering deep into the flower. Therefore, it indicates not just doing things but taking time off to look at others. Strike a balance between work and seeing; not looking – *seeing*.

Butterfly: Despite having a very short life span, butterflies are beautiful insects who are always a delight to see. They are associated with souls in some cultures. A butterfly is also a solid indication of transformation. Its very journey from caterpillar to pupa to butterfly is a magical trek. Some people regard the presence of a butterfly as a sign of someone's marriage, so generally, it is always an excellent insect to see.

Caterpillar: This small insect is slow in its movement and subsists on leaves. It is a symbol of metamorphosis. Certain caterpillars slowly metamorphose into butterflies. That is the message from this tiny creature. This metamorphosis is complete, from caterpillar to butterfly - a total makeover. Therefore, if you see caterpillars repeatedly, then accept it as a message which means that changes have to be made, not cosmetic changes, but profound changes. It is perhaps time to let go of the past and envision a new way of life; in fact, a new future.

Crickets & Grasshoppers: These creatures are generally thought of as bringers of good fortune, and harming them in any way is a no-no. Enjoy their presence - they are not harmful, just playful creatures. Crickets and grasshoppers use their antennae to decode their environment. It is an indication to use the senses differently and connect to the Cosmic Spirit.

Dragonflies: These beautiful insects have the ability to change their flight paths abruptly. This change in direction is the symbol. This shows that alterations in the course you take are sometimes of the essence, especially if the path currently being followed is not going anywhere. The idea is flexibility and the ability to make changes quickly and decisively.

Firefly: This insect carries a light. Its entrance into a home is generally considered auspicious. It gives out the sense of illumination of the spirit. In addition, the firefly is a harbinger of good tidings, including an upcoming marriage.

Fly: This insect is a troublesome one. When it buzzes around, it creates an atmosphere of irritation. However, if flies regularly invade your home, it could be trying to say something. Possibly it means that some aggravating factors in life need to be resolved. This may be a time to let go and make room for new.

Ladybug: It is traditionally said, whenever a ladybug lands on your body, don't flick it away. It is a sign that something you have desired for a long time is coming your way at last. It is also a sign of affection and love.

Mosquitos: These are pesky insects, and most people try to swat them. Yet, the peskiness might mean that certain areas of your life contain irritable elements. Therefore, it is time to remove those minor irritants; the faster, the better. There are many other ideas about mosquitoes, but the most important one is the removal of uncomfortable factors.

Moth: A cousin of the butterfly, in certain cultures, its appearance suggests that the Soul of an ancestor has come to visit. However, moths tend to fly towards light sources, even if that light spells danger. This indicates that not everything that shines is worth having. A movement towards too much materialism is dangerous and counterproductive. Moths being nocturnal, are sometimes thought to be associated with secret and esoteric knowledge.

Spider: Most people do not like spiders. They are creepy critters, but a close examination will show that these bugs have incredible powers. They have the capacity to build a web. The web elements are thin, gossamer-like threads, which the spider secretes, a beautifully engineered item. If a spider becomes your totem creature, then it is time to carefully structure your life and devise solutions to the problems at hand. It is also necessary to keep in mind that there is an indication that you might get stuck in some sort of web without knowing it, so be cautious in your planning.

Wasp: When this insect enters your home, it could be a warning for you. In essence, it is saying that something disagreeable is about to enter the home. It could be a guest or a piece of furniture. Whatever it is, the results may not be favorable. Wasps generally appear when something is about to go wrong. Take heed and keep a close watch on anything about to enter your home. Wasps are involved in pollination; thus, they are symbols of fertility. Keep this important aspect in mind, too!

MORE ON ANIMAL SYMBOLISM

Animal symbolism, while quite potent, is a tricky question to address. The issue is that one does not get a chance to see animals roaming the streets. Instead, they can be seen in zoos, or if lucky, in the wild. Most often, people visit National Parks where animals are protected. Now, going to such a park and seeing animals does not count as an animal symbol for an individual.

Seeing an animal once in the wild could be a sign. If it reappears in dreams, then it is of definite significance. Small animals, such as dogs and cats, are quite common, as we keep them as pets.

Animals, like tigers, are of importance if they appear in dreams. Tigers personify strength and power. They are predators with the ability to plan and catch prey. So, if a tiger is a frequent dream subject, it is trying to tell you to be strong. Lions, too, belong to this category. So, a recurrent dream of lions is a definite sign that the dreamer needs to be stronger and masterful of their lives.

Similarly, elephants may appear in dreams. The elephant is a large animal and is ordinarily peaceful. It is, however, powerful and protective of its young. The truth that the dream is trying to tell you: be strong and protective towards family.

It is necessary to understand whether a sight of an animal is actually a sign or just a sighting. If the animal behaves in some way that denotes that it has a message for you, then, of course, pay attention. This may happen in zoos, too. The trick is to be fully aware and present in reality at all times. However, if spiritual awakening is taking place, this should not be an issue.

Animal symbolism is important and powerful. Therefore, animals constantly appearing in dreams is something to be aware of. The Cosmic Powers are reaching out and trying to offer guidance. Try and understand what it means. Does it indicate a sense of power and strength, as a tiger or a lion does? If so, how does it connect with your reality? Is there something that needs strength to be overcome? Is it something that has become a hurdle for a long time? Time to realign your mental state and act with courage and positivity. It is perhaps the moment when inner fears are to be put aside and allow for a new vision and feeling of power to manifest itself.

Gentler animals, like deer, are symbols of harmony and friendliness. They also represent speed. The deer is a fast animal. Therefore, think of ways to push something ahead with speed but with an attending gentleness and sympathy. This means not hurting anyone else while pushing your agenda.

Several other symbols may be trying to send you a Cosmic message:

Feathers falling at your feet, somewhere close by, or drifting into your room is a sign. Pick up the feather and examine it. Among Native Americans, a feather is considered a sacred symbol. It denotes strength and honor. That's why chiefs and the Braves wore them on their headdresses. The eagle feather was the bestower of a unique dignity. Therefore, feathers are potent symbols. The spirit world may leave feathers for you to see as a way to guide and encourage you. They will catch your attention at a time when you need it. When you see them, think about what you were thinking about at the time of the sighting. Let's see how to decipher their meaning. ***The color of the feather is what needs to be studied.***

- **White** is an indication of purity, spirituality, and the element of serenity. When you see this feather, your angels are watching over and protecting you.
- **Red** is said to represent the Muladhara Chakra in the Indian system of Tantric Yoga. It is the root chakra where the power lies coiled. It is a message that there could be some opportunity coming your way, which is dormant, ready to awaken and make its effects felt.
- **Blue** seems to align with the Vishuddha Chakra in the Tantras, which lies at the throat. This means that you have been truthful and honest in your dealings with the world. The central idea is to carry on.
- **Yellow** is compared to the Manipura Chakra of the Tantras, which is positioned in the solar plexus. This chakra relates to wisdom, joy, and self-control. You are on the right path.
- **Green** is generally associated with growth, emotions, healing, and love.
- **Orange** is a color that indicates a sense of confidence and sensuality.
- **Pink** signifies compassion, assisting others, and the importance of giving in general.
- **Grey** is a neutral color and represents neutrality and flexibility.
- **Purple** is sometimes compared to the Sahasrara Chakra of the Tantras. The Crown Chakra. It signifies that the connection with the Divine is in the offing and that the universal consciousness is close.
- **Brown** is a color that announces connections to the Earth. But, grounded as it were to the Earth, it also means solidity.

- **Black** is usually associated with a sense of transformation. It also denotes hidden activities and new insight.

Different cultures, especially the ancient ones, have their own interpretations of these symbols. As a matter of fact, interpretations work best when the individual circumstances are considered. Using the guide presented here, think of how it represents your current state. Be flexible in your thoughts. The interpretations are not rigid but just a basic indication of the symbol's meaning. Sit in meditation, and see what message you receive. Ancient symbolism and meaning lie deep in the unconscious. It is best when trying to analyze sightings of animals, birds, insects, and feathers to not try and read into them using your conscious mind. That will never reveal the real nature of the symbol. Symbols are more than their appearance. Let the sighting sink into your mind and slowly descend into the unconscious. The unconscious, the root matter, will send you the answer. It is beyond the powers of the conscious mind to read such symbols.

Sometimes, a particular tune might awaken memories that were lying buried inside you. This is also a signal that you are perhaps ready for something. At all times, remember not to fixate on things with your conscious mind. It is your unconscious that is the key.

Chapter 5
Intuition, Consciousness, and the Subconsciousness

To understand what spiritual awakening is all about, a little knowledge regarding the structure of the mind is necessary. We are talking about the Conscious mind, the Subconscious mind, and their relation to the faculty of intuition. All three are connected. They function in tandem, as it were. But, first, we deal with the Conscious mind.

The conscious mind is the one we are aware of all the time. It is that part of the mind which regulates our daily actions and feelings. It enables us to function, perceive and hear things, creating visual and audio images that the brain retains as memory. It is what controls our movements and thoughts on a personal level. It is also the filter that prevents the subconscious mind from invading our conscious thoughts and feelings. Therefore, it is the most visible and known part of the mind. It is, in fact, the top layer of the mind; just below it is the subconscious. The conscious mind processes data from our sense perceptions, and the brain then uses the data as it comes through. That is why people say they have consciously decided to do this or that. This is because they are acting through the conscious portion of the brain.

"Most people confuse 'self-knowledge' with knowledge of their ego-personalities," wrote C. G. Jung in his essay entitled, "The Undiscovered Self." He explains that anyone who has ego-consciousness thinks he knows himself, but this is intrinsically a mistaken view. It is here that we come to the subconscious. The ego knows only its own contents and not those of the subconscious, which Jung refers to as the 'unconscious.' Right here is the issue at hand. The subconscious mind, although it exists in everyone, is not known. The conscious mind has control. An average person measures his knowledge by what his environment is telling him. He totally ignores the real, physical facts that exist. He is, in fact, unaware of them.

Self-knowledge is, therefore, a restrictive kind of knowledge, limited in scope and depth. Nevertheless, the subconscious mind is always at work. In his study of the unconscious, Freud became aware that strange forces lurked in the subconscious. He was afraid that these were of an opaque nature and decided not to mention them. Freud was right. There are forces of an enigmatic nature residing within the subconscious. It is these forces that an inward meditative exercise can bring up. It is, in one way, the Primordial Soul of the Universe, something in which we all share.

To ignore the subconscious is to allow it to interact with the conscious mind and raise issues that may not be favorable. There are dark areas in there, too. People often say that such a terrible thing has never happened before in their family. How, then, to explain the terrible happening? The erroneous judgment is based on knowledge of the conscious Self, and the subconscious has not been considered. It is necessary to consider the subconscious, for it contains the root matter.

It is known that the unconscious (subconscious) contains suppressed memories or thoughts, some not pleasant. As they do not disappear, these submerged memories remain and may emerge with devastating consequences over time. The mind at the second level is just below the conscious mind but just as powerful.

The word 'unconscious' will be used instead of 'subconscious' from now on, as they mean the same thing.

That great psychic powers exist in the unconscious is not debated anymore. The problem is tapping into them without letting loose dark and damaging content. This is why someone might do something dramatic after leading a peaceful life, which is dramatically opposed to his known character. This is the effect of the unconscious showing up in the conscious mind, making the event happen. The person has really no idea from where that terrible instinct came.

In some cases, the person, when questioned, appears dazed and confused and cannot offer any coherent explanation for his actions. The authorities, in all countries, can testify to this. He cannot explain his behavior because he does not know from where the urge came. It came from his unconscious, something about which he has no clue.

Typically, the unconscious stays out of sight. The ego controls the conscious mind, which everyone sees and knows, but the unconscious sends messages to the conscious mind, influencing our decisions and actions. We are just not aware of it. It is not the intention to completely subdue the ego, which could lead to results that aren't ideal. What spiritual awakening means is to reduce the power of the ego so that the unconscious can surface with the contents which are real - the actual Self. This is what is the main aim of meditation. When we look inward, the senses are no longer distracted by external stimuli. These external stimuli are a barrier to any psychic development. They are like loud sounds, which suffocate the inner voice, which needs to be heard. This voice comes from the unconscious. It is where the Primal image of the Self resides. That is the Self with which we want to get in touch. It is the authentic Self. In cooperation with the conscious mind, our ego has created a Self that we feel we know. A spiritual awakening is a process to get in touch with the real you!

The meditation process will slowly alert the unconscious mind to surface and the ego to take a backseat. After a while, the ego accepts the influence of the unconscious. It is aware that a new self is being created. This is the new you, in touch with your inner reality. The ego, then, will not try and dominate your life completely, as it has been in the habit of doing. The cessation of external stimuli reduces the power of the ego.

How do we know that the unconscious mind is being heard? ***Be prepared for some dark stuff to surface, initially.*** This is material that the unconscious contains along with many other thoughts and memories, some of which are good. It is the unconscious telling you that it is in operation. As mentioned earlier, these thoughts must be allowed to play out. After these have had their share, the real Self will slowly begin to appear. This can be in the form of images, visions, signs, and symbols - things that you have never seen before.

It is, however, advisable to proceed slowly. If it is negated or made dysfunctional, the ego could lead to undesirable consequences. That is why the system provided in this book is safe. It leads to steady and continuous progress towards spiritual awakening.

What now begins to happen is that the Ego Self is slowly modified. It is seen as a mental construct that is not real and created by the ego and the conscious mind. This realization is of immense importance. In the beginning, this may appear confusing. But just go with what the unconscious is doing. It will reveal the truth, never fear. Then, you will know intuitively at some point that what is happening is spiritual. The question then arises: how do I know that my intuition is working? To answer that, you need to know what 'intuition' is, where it comes from, and how it operates.

The word 'intuition' comes from the word 'intueri,' which means "to look into or upon." The power of intuition is commonly known. Everyone, at some time or other, has felt its action. It is a power that resides in the unconscious, as far as is known. The reason is easy to see. You cannot say that I will now have an intuitive insight or vision. It doesn't work that way. In fact, it comes when the mind is distracted and not focussed on something. It is clear that the conscious mind has no control over it, and therefore, does not arise from it.

Intuition is a psychological function of the unconscious. It unconsciously transmits perceptions. This perception can be about external or internal objects or their association with something. This perception is neither sensation nor feeling, nor intellectual conclusion, although it may appear in any of these forms. The subject of the intuitive revelation appears as a whole without any explanation of where it came from. It is somewhat like an instinctive feeling that just presents the feeling. It is not a sensation, nor has it a rational basis. This does not mean that it is not trying to reveal something. Quite the opposite, but the problem is that it does not offer explanatory notes.

Let us examine what intuition can do and how it manifests itself suddenly without warning. Here is what the mathematician Henri Poincare said about intuitive knowledge:

"These sudden inspirations are never produced....except after some days of voluntary efforts which appeared absolutely fruitless, in which one thought one had accomplished nothing and seemed to be on a wrong track. These efforts however were not as barren as one thought; they set the unconscious machine in motion, and without them it would not have worked at all."

(From The Imprisoned Splendour - Raynor C. Johnson - 1977)

Poincare is talking about the intuitive flash of revelation, which derives from the unconscious. This is the inspiration about which he is talking. Intuition has always produced revelations of significant kinds.

One of the founders of organic chemistry, August Kekule, sitting idly without any particular thought in mind, in a sort of somnolent state, is said to have suddenly had a vision of a snake eating its own tail. At this time, he was working on the structure of Benzene. This sudden vision told him that the structure was ring-shaped. It was.

An intuitive flash of inspiration had given him the answer for which he was looking.

Henri Bergson, a renowned French philosopher, studied psychic events and the unconscious. He always gave more importance to the intuitive faculty of the mind than the conscious one, where the apprehension of reality was concerned. He believed that the intuitive faculty gave reality a far more accurate picture. The rational conscious mind could never reach the depths which the unconscious could.

How can an intuitive flash be identified? It is necessary to think carefully. What did the flash of insight make you feel? Usually, the thought or feeling just comes out of nowhere. It may have signified that the party you plan to go to tonight might not turn out well for you. Well, the best way would be to go to the party and test the reality of the flash. You will be surprised when you find that for certain unexplained reasons, the party didn't go well for you at all. So, your intuition was spot on!

As you develop your spiritual awakening, these will slowly become more and more common. You have connected to a power that is providing you with guidance. Since intuitive flashes are not explanatory, you may have to figure out what they mean. Sometimes, these messages do not seem to have any coherence. That's because the unconscious does not work rationally and linearly that our conscious mind does. Remember, however, that you cannot control this faculty. It works at its own will. Most good astrologers will tell you that, sometimes, they are not aware of how they arrived at a particular prediction. This is because the unconscious worked so quickly that the entire process was too fast for the conscious mind to comprehend. That was intuition in action! It is well known in astrology that the Moon, which rules our thoughts, if in a water sign - Pisces, Cancer, Scorpio - then it gives the person the power of intuition built-in. It just needs to be developed. The depth of the water is akin to the depth of the unconscious.

Dealing with intuition isn't very tough. Initially, you may not get it, literally. Yet, if you keep all your senses alert, you will begin to identify intuitive insights. You suddenly get a feeling or premonition that something is going to happen. You have no idea what or where. Just stay calm, and observe what does happen. It may not be close to you, but something will happen. Once the event takes place, you will know what your intuition tells you. The point is that the flashes are not always very detailed. They are sometimes just a feeling, a quick sensation of some fact.

Let's look at another example. You are in a park, by yourself. It is, let's say, 5 p.m. You plan to leave at six and be home by six-thirty. Suddenly, you get a feeling that you must get home. You rise and get home by five-thirty to find that everything is normal. Did that intuitive message lie to you? Now, here's the thing. Check what happens between five-thirty and when you had initially planned to come back: six-thirty. What has happened in that one hour that you would have missed if you had come back as usual? Did an important phone call come? Did someone you haven't seen for ages suddenly drop in? Or did somebody in the house need your help? You will indeed find something you would have missed had you come back later. It is necessary to analyze these things carefully. Not every intuitive flash is about earth-shattering events.

Intuition is sometimes like ESP (Extrasensory Perception). This is now accepted even by scientists. Several studies have shown that some people do possess ESP. This is akin to an intuitive feeling about something. Sometimes, it is difficult to tell the difference.

When driving a car, something inside you tells you to be careful. So take heed and watch out. These feelings are most often intuitive events warning you ahead of time.

Now is the time to address an important issue: **the difference between thinking and intuition.** It is necessary to understand the difference so that you don't confuse conscious thinking with intuition.

Thinking is essentially a conscious operation with the backing of the ego. It is basically linear in design. That means when a person thinks he is taking bits and pieces of thought and trying to form a coherent whole or trying to figure out where the bits and pieces fit. There is always a cause-and-effect element in this kind of thinking. The ego has its own two bits in it. This compartmentalized view of things affects how our mind works - the conscious mind, that is! Thinking means when a person is using his conscious mind to work out something.

On the other hand, intuition does not think; it just is. That means that when you get an intuitive feeling, it has no rationale behind the thought – it makes you feel something. It is the whole thought. There is no before or after, just one sensation, and that's it. Since it comes from the unconscious, it can sometimes be a powerful feeling. Verbal cues are not present. What it wants to say is a sudden and intense surge of feeling. It comes and is gone in a second. There are no clues as to where it came from or where it went, and unlike conscious thinking, it offers no explanation.

Therefore, thinking is what you consciously do. Intuition is what you receive without asking. You receive this primarily when the conscious mind is not working or is at rest. It is when the mind is at rest that intuition appears. It is, remember, the product of the unconscious. The fact that the one works when the other doesn't is proof enough that they are separate entities.

Conscious thinking is what we do all the time. Going out, shopping, going to work, etc., are all conscious decisions backed by thinking. The intuitive faculty never comes to the forefront except in infrequent circumstances during these times. The mind is too caught up with the minutiae of life. The mind is in an agitated state, and intuition is quiet.

'I have to leave now to catch my flight. It will take me an hour to reach the airport.' These are examples of thinking. They are lateral, cause and effect. If you do not leave on time, you will miss the flight.

If there is some peace and quiet in between, the intuition might send a feeling of danger. If such a feeling is strong, it is wise to listen to it. It is sometimes difficult to differentiate between an intuitive feeling and just a feeling of fright. The latter must be overcome, and the former must be adequately heard.

The question will inevitably arise as to how to increase this intuitive faculty. Well, the unconscious is a funny thing. It cannot always be told what to do. In fact, it is almost impossible to do so! With that in mind, what is to be done? The first thing to do is allow periods of silence when the conscious mind is quiet. That means not thinking about life's mundane matters and giving the mind a rest. This is best done through meditation. If meditation is properly carried on, the mind begins to quiet down slowly, and the rush of thoughts winds down. It is then that the unconscious can be heard. Meditation also helps the unconscious become more active and the ego-controlled conscious mind to slow down. It is when the mind is unoccupied that intuition works. Enlightenment occurs during intense meditation. That is the way our minds are constructed. Although nobody fully understands the mysterious workings of the brain, some facts seem to be accepted.

Another way to increase the power of the unconscious is by using your whole being to feel the universe around you. Some sensations abound and need to be noticed and felt. These feelings drop down into the unconscious. The conscious mind does not deal with them, as it is solely the province of the unconscious. Once you practice doing this, your unconscious will start responding. Intuition becomes more and more active.

Since it arises from the unconscious, the intuitive faculty can only be improved by connecting with the unconscious. Therefore, there are no direct ways of doing this. The only way is through developing your meditative techniques, sense of awareness, and connection to the Cosmic Source.

The more you allow your inner self to speak, the more the intuitive faculty will come into play. It is the inner voice. The conscious mind and the ego need to be controlled to allow this voice to be heard. This does not mean that the inner voice sends out verbal cues. It means that it changes aspects of your mind. These are changes that you can feel but not actively understand. Slowly, though, you will become aware that certain changes are taking place.

Once these changes start happening, your perceptions of life will undergo modification. Your view will become more understanding. You will feel less angry and depressed when things don't go your way. This means that there will be an increased sense of equilibrium in your life. Unfortunately, the average person today does not have that balance. Their thoughts resemble a roller coaster ride, where emotions and actions keep going up and down. This affects their lives adversely. Meditation and awareness slow down the roller coaster. The thing is to get off the bumpy ride and maintain equilibrium in your thoughts and actions.

With this connection, it is important to pay attention to your dreams. **Dreams come from the unconscious, and therefore, are of great importance.** Dreams sometimes bring forth your deepest desires and sometimes tell you which way your life is going. If you carefully study your dreams, you can, when necessary, take corrective action. It is, however, not necessary to worry about dreams all the time. That is a negative way of handling things. Just be aware of them and their message.

Creativity of any kind helps the unconscious speak up. For example, it is a good idea to draw, put together a scrapbook, or even keep a journal. These activities tend to help look inward and give the unconscious a chance to work. Remember, all great artists - especially painters - used this power. Their ideas nearly always involved the unconscious.

It is known that great scientists, like Richard Feynman, went to their country retreats for inspiration. They walked around amidst nature in silence. Why do you think they would do that? The reason is simple: solitude and the ability to hear their inner voice. The other reason is that nature speaks as part of the great Cosmic Spirit. Mystics everywhere are aware of this. Poets, too, are familiar with this power. The poets Shelley and Yeats admitted that sometimes they just wrote poetry guided by an unknown hand – that the poem just appeared out of nowhere! That was the unconscious doing its stuff!

Therefore, walking in the woods or areas with few people is a great way to feel your unconscious mind. Thoughts and ideas manifest themselves without any effort on your part. It is necessary to get past the mundane and the ordinary. This is only possible through an enhanced sense of perception, something which only the unconscious can bring to the table.

There is less interference from artificial energy levels created by electricity and RF signals in places like the forest or the mountains, which power our mobile phones. These interfere with the vibrations of the body. It is necessary to get out of their range as far as possible sometimes to enable the unconscious to act. Do that as many times as you can.

Another way to increase intuition is to see how it worked for you before you embarked on this path to awakening. Think back to events in your own life. Did you get some kind of warning or premonition at the time? Sit alone, and carefully go back in time. Was there what is called a "gut feeling" present? If there was, that was intuition warning you. What people call "gut feelings" are also messages from the unconscious, which have a physical presence. The feeling is real. The conscious mind has latched onto the intuitive feeling generated by the unconscious and turned it into a physical symptom. What you need to analyze is what you did then. Did you listen to your gut feeling? Or did you ignore it? Was the gut feeling correct in predicting the outcome of the event? That is a clue that gave you bursts of intuition. If you had a gut feeling every time, then understand that the path of awakening you have now chosen was already indicated.

The body, too, is affected by intuition. Pay attention when you sense that something inside is trying to tell you something. Is that feeling causing heaviness and discomfort in the body physically? Or is it driving lightness and exhilaration? If the former, then take care. Examine your proposed decision or action carefully to look for alternative solutions. Again, the unconscious is sending you an alert.

Daily life is a web that people are caught up in constantly. It is most often stressful and leaves little time to think of other things - the things that really matter! This daily grind exhausts the mind and the body. A great idea would be to just get away for a bit to a place where you are free just to be idle. By idle, I mean resting your mind, detached from the travails of daily life, and as a popular saying goes, "resting your Soul." It is one of the best medicines to rejuvenate your mind and body. What it can do is get the unconscious to work. A good way is to disengage the conscious mind.

Some psychologists call the unconscious the "shadow mind" and say that you must engage with it. Not doing so could lead to unfavorable consequences. This shadow mind contains all our secrets, things we wish to keep hidden. Psychology calls them "repressed memories."

Even when you are away from everything, your conscious mind will continue to engage your thoughts with the affairs of daily life, bringing to the forefront problems and issues that need to be resolved. It isn't easy to get rid of them, but here is a way to do this. Sit quietly in a location where your vision travels over an open space. It could be the ocean. In cities, vision is blocked by buildings and structures and can travel a short distance, but the ability to let your eyes travel over a long distance has value. Now that your vision is looking at nothing in particular, but is in a way looking at an infinite distance, try and think of some piece of music which you really like. Think of the tune, and let it play in your head. Don't focus on anything else. Basically, let your mind wander. A feeling of peace will slowly descend. The unconscious is elevating a part of the inner voice. With practice, you will come to recognize that feeling and want it often. It is quite possible that you may have a vision of something beautiful. Enjoy it!

This self-empowerment is something at which you alone will need to work. It is your personal journey. Positivity and a sense of awareness, a belief that you are part of something beautiful and transcendent, is what will slowly color your life and make mundane things superficial. It will teach you to let go.

Chapter 6
Purpose

What is my purpose in life? This is an important but difficult question to answer analytically. Over many centuries, sages have been discussing this. They have laid out certain facts which are relevant to this question. Let's look at those for a start.

The philosophies of the East view life as a journey, with each birth being a part of this journey. Ancient Western philosophies, too, say the same thing. Socrates, in his dialogues, enters into the discussion of the immortality of the Soul. So, the Greeks, too, were aware of it. But what does all of this mean?

Let's start at the beginning - birth. A child is born into a particular family and inherits half the father's DNA and half the mother's DNA. They, however, get the mitochondrial DNA solely from their mother. Therefore, they are born in circumstances that were not of their choosing, if truth be told. The family's economic circumstances will, to an extent, decide their initial life. Not all of it, but the major portion of their childhood. If they are born into a wealthy family, they will have the best that the world can offer. If in a low-income family, they will make do as best they can.

That said, **what is the purpose of birth** in each case? The boy/girl born in an affluent family will probably live in the lap of luxury unless circumstances take a turn for the worse somewhere down the line. On the other hand, the boy/girl born in straitened circumstances will inevitably have to struggle.

This is the basic fact of life. It would appear that the purpose of life is to work and enjoy all the offerings as much as possible, circumstances permitting. However, as mystics will tell you, this is a blinkered view of life, one which is surrounded by illusion. A life in which happiness and tragedy will appear makes life sometimes easy and sometimes difficult and worrisome. A rich man has a luxurious life but does not necessarily follow his joy. His worries are significant, and great wealth brings great concern.

So, where do we go from here? Well, we consider what the mystics have to say to get a handle on what is the purpose of life. First, each Soul is reborn in specific circumstances to play out its role in that birth. The law of Karma states this quite clearly.

The Soul of the child who is born brings with it the consequences of the child's previous incarnations. Typically, no one remembers their previous lives. Yet, some do, and there are currently documented cases where people remember parts of their past life. Usually, however, people are prevented from remembering their past lives by the Cosmic Power. In the Bhagavad Gita, Krishna famously tells Arjun that while he remembers all his past lives, Arjun cannot. Krishna is a divine being in human form, and therefore, privy to the Divine secrets. Knowing one's past lives could make human life difficult, hence the veil placed over it.

The whole concept of 'purpose' is the issue. It isn't just about enjoying yourself. It has a far deeper purpose, something which the veil of Maya hides from most people, until and unless the person begins questioning their reason for existing. That's the beginning of the inward journey. In fact, the beginning of wisdom, as the ancients say, "If thou seekest me, thou hast found me!"

The real purpose of birth as a human being is to realize the Cosmic Divine and move to become one with it. That is the ultimate goal, but it cannot be reached easily. So when a desire for spiritual awakening makes itself felt, the person, without knowing it, is actually desirous of union with the Godhead. That's what is at the core of it - nothing else.

It starts with a sense of disquiet, desire for solitude, and a moving away from the vicissitudes of everyday life. It is the beginning of the subliminal longing for the Divine. That is the purpose of life - the real purpose. This is not to say that everyone should be busy meditating and becoming a hermit. The fact is not everyone gets this desire. It happens to a select few. This is decided on the Soul's journey through previous incarnations and the Karma associated with it. So, if you desire a spiritual awakening, you are, in fact, ready for it. The need makes itself felt only when the person is ready to make the journey. Consider yourself a blessed person!

There are ways to feel more purposeful. Start by being generous. Give back to society some of what you got from it. Help those in need, financial or otherwise. Give to those who need aid. Help a colleague get through difficult times. These are some of the acts which can make life more purposeful. Generosity and benevolence towards humanity are among the most satisfying pleasures in life. The fact of the matter is that it is perhaps the thing that satisfies and generates an enormous sense of purpose. Life becomes meaningful. Therefore, practice as much generosity as you can. You are, in fact, building up good Karma. The effects will begin to rub off on you. A sense that you are connected to humanity is a terrific feeling.

The mystic purpose is, of course, connecting with the Divine. That is the highest purpose of Man. However, that is a long journey. Spiritual awakening is just the beginning but an essential beginning. It means that you are on the path already, which is very important. To become more connected to the Cosmic forces is an excellent direction in which to be heading. The journey should add to your feeling of a meaningful life.

People suffer from the loss of individuality and a sense of disorientation as to their role in life. This leaves them with a continuous sense of unhappiness. Called in ancient times a "loss of soul." Modern man feels that he is a tiny, insignificant cog in a giant machine, which he can neither see in its entirety nor understand the purpose. This feeling of insignificance is the cause of a lot of mental unhappiness. This makes people feel the absence of any kind of purpose. That is until they get to understand, to know that they are all part of the same symphony and that no one is smaller or bigger. This needs to be understood.

The best way is to take a step back from life and see what it is all about. The answer is there; you just have to see it. Just ask yourself whether you were born to get to work, go to the club, come back, eat, sleep (with a bit of telly in between), and repeat the same thing day in and day out? Sounds rather bland and dull? It is actually both. It is necessary to get connected to something to feel purposeful, something which can remove the feeling of restlessness and insignificance. Giving and lending a helping hand is one way. Another is to do something creative. Start learning to play piano, guitar, or whatever instrument you like. Music unlocks a different part of the brain. It will start coloring your life, giving it beauty and meaning; the perception of beauty is an integral part of life. If you feel you don't have it, start developing it immediately. This sense of beauty does not mean that you just say, "Oh, the roses are lovely!". That's not it at all. Until you feel the beauty speak to you and something inside responds, you haven't got it yet. Your senses must respond. There is receiving and sending, which needs to happen. Painters who worked on landscapes knew this. They would visually speak to nature. You won't get the real feel of nature, otherwise. Nature is miserly in that way; it will unveil its secrets only to a genuine admirer. **Ultimately, do what brings you joy and a sense of connection!**

Talk to people you know and to people you meet. A few leading questions will tell you that they are not really happy with their lives. If you listen carefully, discontent will show up. They may bluster about how happy they are and how they recently bought a new house and so on. After a while, they will reveal their feelings truthfully. Not all people are unhappy, of course. Some people are content in the truest sense of the word. Why are they happy? What do they do that makes them happy? The chances are that they are doing something which they love to do. They are also engaged in trying to help people in their own way. For example, they could be making sure that their family feels loved and taken care of. These they do unconsciously. They are generally outgoing and always willing to lend a hand. They express positive vibrations and spread them among people they meet. This gives them a purpose in life! That's why they are happy.

Now, spiritual awakening is a process that works from the inside. You can help it along by using the same technique used by the content people. A purpose in life boosts the spirit, and the spiritual awakening actually happens quicker.

Find a way where your new, intuitive feelings can assist those in need. Use your newfound skills to reach out. Remember, you have a deeper understanding of things now, and this will only get deeper as the days go on. It is a gift, so use it wisely!

We now come to an important subject: the meaning of numbers in your life. Numbers, as the ancients knew, were not just 'numbers' but a sign of mystical phenomena, too. The Kabbalah of Numbers uses numbers to chart the destiny of people. Each number has a value, and each number has a specific function.

The regular appearance of specific numbers in your life means that the Cosmos is trying to send you a message. It could be telling you that you are on the right path, or it could be telling you to change your direction. In either case, the numbers mean something. Numerology, especially the Kabbalah of Numbers, mentions each number from 0 to 9 as significant. Each number is ruled by a planet, the same ones used in astrology. All these systems say the same thing at the base, and their message seems to mesh magically. If one looks at the Cosmic significance of numbers, certain indications are worth noting. There are what are called "Angel Numbers," which have been part of your life consistently. These numbers are your guide. They are numerical messages sent by the Cosmos. Sometimes, these numbers have to do with your life path number, and these numbers are present in some way during significant events in life, like marriage, the birth of children, first job, and so on. They are always uncannily present. Coincidence? Nothing's a coincidence! **There is energy in numbers and a mystical side to them. The ancient Greeks knew about this. The most renowned of them is Pythagoras.**

House and street numbers are most likely to appear as numbers familiar to you. This is because they are quite astonishingly related to your life path number. Check this out for yourself. It's bizarre, but it is how the Cosmos works, and few ever realize this. They don't even notice the appearance of these recurring numbers in their lives. However, once you are on the path to spiritual awakening, your awareness of these messages will slowly become evident. As your awareness increases, you will see them automatically. It won't be necessary to go around looking for them actively. Instead, the Cosmos will direct your attention to them when the need arises.

This portion of the chapter is meant to give you a basic understanding of your life path number and Angel Numbers. For more on this, please refer to the author's book, "The Spiritual Meanings of Numbers."

When finding your purpose in life, a significant number is your life path number. This will reveal your strengths and weaknesses, among other things, which will aid you on your journey. **You can focus on your gifts to find purpose in your life and know the areas that need work.** It is arrived at by adding a person's birth date. As previously discussed, this is done as follows:

- Date of Birth: 16.6.2005 - 16th becomes 1+6=7. Then, the month is added: 7+6=13. Then, we add the year digits together: 2+0+0+5

= 7. We now add this '7' to the previous '13'. We get 20, which is reduced by adding 2+0=2. Therefore, the life path number is '2'.

This number will always play an essential part in your life. Once you become aware of its importance, you will notice its presence regularly in your journey through life.

The spiritual significance of the numbers 0 to 9 are as follows:

- THE NUMBER 'ZERO'
  - This number is associated with the planet **Pluto** and with the star sign **Scorpio.** In the Tarot, it is associated with "The Fool."
  - *The Major Message of this number: "Continue to do what you are doing."*
  - **Zero** represents infinity or the pure spirit that knows no beginning or end. It is the cyclic process of birth and rebirth. It also means the 'Void' or nothing. This is where the Pure Spirit resides. It is a sign which indicates spirituality or oneness with the Great Consciousness. If it appears with another number, say the number 60, it enhances and empowers the number '6'. It is, in effect, saying to pay attention to the number '6'. When the number appears as zero, then it means you need to stick to your path.

- THE NUMBER 'ONE'

  - This number is associated with the **Sun** and the star sign **Aries**. In the Tarot, it is The Sun/The Magician.
  - The colors of this number are Red/Yellow.
  - The Letters associated are A, J, S.
  - *The Major Message of this number: "Move forward with belief. Success is yours."*
  - The number One indicates individualistic people. They want to find their own way, and they have to face alienation and loneliness. Success, however, is assured if the path is followed relentlessly.

- The personality of people with the number **One** is confident and independent. Their weaknesses are ego, overconfidence, and stubbornness.
- They can be insensitive to the needs and feelings of others. These negative traits need to be addressed if progress is to be made.
- People with this number find it difficult to be in relationships. Their attitude of independence and stubbornness can lead to problems with others. A fixed mindset is not a very desirable one. It leads to trouble. In the workplace, the appearance of the number **One** means that the Cosmos wants you to develop a more cooperative state of mind.
- **Angel Number ONE** means, "Work with others and move forward. Time to begin something new."

- The Number **TWO**

  - This number is associated with the **Moon**. In the Tarot, it is The Moon/The High Priestess.
  - The colors of this number are Orange/Blue.
  - The Letters associated are B, K, T.
  - *The Major Message of this number: "Considering the depth of relationships."*
  - The number Two indicates a person who is a healer and a mediator for peace. The main idea is to develop and maintain a harmonious world.
  - The basic personality is compassionate, non-judgmental, honest, responsible, and friendly. These people are soft at heart, but they must learn to stand up for themselves sometimes. They must also develop the ability not to be swayed by everything or everybody.
  - The number **Two** indicates a need for self-expression in the workplace, which external forces must not hamper. Since working in highly stressful environments does not suit this number, it is necessary to avoid such places as much as possible.

- This number, being ruled by the **Moon,** gives a strong sense of intuition. Therefore, it is a valuable tool and should be utilized often.
- It is necessary to exercise caution in personal relationships and not be swayed by emotions.

- The Number **THREE**

  - This number is associated with the planet Jupiter. The star sign is Gemini.
  - The color of this number is Yellow.
  - The associated Letters are C, I, U.
  - ***The Major Message of this number: "Release what you are holding back."***
  - The individuals with this number as their life path number are afraid to express themselves. They need to open up and work towards their goals, not hold back. Focus on doing due diligence - that is the secret.
  - People with this number are friendly, independent, and, if they try, expressive. In addition, they have excellent communication skills and a solid sense of intuition.
  - If they want to, they can manipulate people easily. That is something they should beware of, as manipulating people invariably backfires.
  - The main issues are; that they are hesitant at expressing themselves and their inability to stick to their jobs. The **Three** energy tends to make them job-hoppers.
  - The number **Three** has a special significance as it is the Holy Trinity, and this may mean that Higher Souls are acting as spirit guides. Therefore, special attention needs to be paid when the number Three appears. It is essentially a sacred number.

- The Number **FOUR**

  - This number is associated with the planet **Uranus** and the star sign **Taurus.** In the Tarot, it is The Emperor.
  - The color of the number is Green.

- Associated Letters: D, M, V.
- *The Major Message of this number: "Take care of the essentials, and with perseverance, all odds will be overcome."*
- People with this number are practical and responsible. They build trust in others, but they could feel trapped or confined by responsibilities undertaken.
- These people are enthusiastic, productive, and somewhat family-oriented. However, they find it challenging to overcome obstacles and give in to self-defeat and martyrdom.
- In the workplace, it may indicate that it is a good idea to be working with smaller teams and work with determination.
- In personal relationships, this number tends to make people care for their loved ones and are dependable and steady. However, it is a good idea for these people to accept the imperfections of others.
- It is necessary to mention here that the number **Four**, which in some numerology systems, represents difficulties and other problems. It is the exact half of the number '8', which is ruled by Saturn and is known to create problems in life. Saturn is the planet of constriction. However, for the purposes of Western thought, this is not considered bad; rather, as a call to perseverance and hard work.

- The Number **FIVE**

  - This number is associated with the planet **Jupiter** and the star sign **Leo**. In the Tarot, it is The Hierophant.
  - The color of this number is Blue.
  - Associated Letters: E, N, W.
  - *The Major Message of this number: "Time to transform."*
  - This number indicates that the person is adventurous and looking for a change.
  - These people generally are individualistic, positive, and adaptable. They typically value personal freedom. However, too much change does not develop any long-term, permanent

relationships. There is a tendency to take on more than one can chew.
- The appearance of **Five** means there is a movement towards a transformation, whether in the person's personal life or the workplace.
- There is a tendency to do everything in excess, and there is a danger of getting into some form of substance abuse. A careful channeling of these energies in the right direction can work well.
- This number may indicate that it is time to re-evaluate current relationships in personal life. If they turn out to be toxic, then it's time to move on.
- The number **Five** corresponds to the five senses, and it is a significant number in esoteric lore.

- The Number **SIX**

  - This number is associated with the planet **Venus** and the star sign **Virgo**. In the Tarot, it is The Lovers.
  - The colors of this number are Indigo/Purple/Green.
  - Associated Letters: F, O, X.
  - ***The Major Message of this number: "It is time to reassess life's daily routine."***
  - There is a tendency to indulge in excess of self-sacrifice with this number. While helping out is always a beneficial activity, overdoing it is harmful.
  - The person is dependable, generous, and caring, but there is a tendency to be bossy at times.
  - It is necessary to balance everything so that life can be pleasant and interesting. However, a tilt towards any extremes may create anxiety and other mental health issues.
  - With the appearance of **Six**, the Cosmos is trying to say that it is time to build communities. This number provides stability. It is this stability that needs to be used.
  - However, this sign is also a warning when it shows itself. It is saying that there is a need to see how the person is handling responsibilities, whether a balance exists between personal and

work-life. If there is, changes need to be made urgently. Learn to say 'no' so that extraneous things do not deflect or complicate life and make suitable changes in relationships so that unhealthy compromises are not required.

- The Number **SEVEN**

    - This number is associated with **Saturn** and the star sign **Libra**. In the Tarot, it is The Chariot
    - The colors of this number are Violet/Purple/Grey. Associated Letters: G, P, Y.
    - *The Major Message of this number: "Time to align with the Divine purpose."*
    - The number **Seven** is considered a magic number and has great significance. It symbolizes spiritual matters and indicates a need to change direction, heading towards a more spiritually oriented goal.
    - Persons ruled by this number are generally philosophically inclined, but a sense of passive acceptance of the world is a significant drawback.
    - In personal life, the person must always be aware of how relationships are going. Philosophical outlooks can sometimes lead to woolly-headed behavior. This is because the heads of such persons are always in the clouds. A more earthy anchor is needed as a soulmate to provide reality and stability.
    - This number always hints at a spirit guide lending a helping hand. The trick is to understand the assistance being provided.

- The Number **EIGHT**

    - This number is associated with **Saturn** and the North Node of The Moon. The star sign is **Leo**. In the Tarot, it is Strength.
    - The color of this number is Silver.
    - Associated Letters: H, Q, Z.
    - *The Major Message of this number: "You have the ability to overcome. Do it".*

- This number often indicates obstacles and difficulties. However, **Eight** also gives the power to overcome those obstacles. It is a journey of learning.
- Hard work brings attendant success, but care must be exercised so that the desire for material success does not obscure the spiritual needs and personal relationships.
- When this number appears in your workplace, it signifies that hurdles are coming. This could be a minor adversity or a serious one. The battle to overcome these leads to an understanding of the spiritual side of life.
- This number makes a person tenacious and gives the willpower to succeed.

- The Number **NINE**

  - This number is associated with the planet **Uranus** and the South Node of the Moon. The star sign is **Sagittarius**. In the Tarot, it is The Hermit.
  - Associated color: Gold.
  - Associated Letters: I, R.
  - ***The Major message of this number: "Love yourself and also others."***
  - Persons who vibrate to this number tend to try and improve the world and make it a better place in which to live. However, there is also a tendency to be arrogant and pushy. This is to be consciously avoided.
  - The individuals with this number are cheerful and charismatic. They are also compassionate human beings.
  - At times, they may appear lazy and disconnected from everything, but that is a temporary phenomenon. They will soon be back.
  - The appearance of **Nine** in the workplace indicates that some sort of difficulty may appear. However, the number gives the power to overcome.
  - It is a number, which, when multiplied by any number and the digits of the answer are added up, amount to **Nine**.

- **Nine** is a mystical number since it is the Trinity multiplied by three.

Now that you understand your life path number and what it means when it appears, it is necessary to look at what are called "Angel Numbers." These numbers are important, and their appearance is always significant.

It is necessary to mention here that recognizing the different Angel Numbers, which tend to come into people's lives, is an extensive subject. A detailed explanation of these matters is found in the author's book, "The Spiritual Meanings of Numbers." Here, we briefly mention a few examples, with a guide to break down complex numbers to follow.

Angel Numbers often appear as triple digits, but they can be single, double, or quadruple. They may appear as repeating numbers or as a number combination. The sure sign is that you will notice them, and they will show up in your life, time and time again. Numbers have energy and are used to grab our attention to encourage and guide us.

Let us start with the number ZERO.

The Number Zero, while by itself, represents nothingness and wholeness and can increase the power of numbers. Consider this: if there is a zero after the number '2' or '3', it becomes 20 or 30, a number of higher value. This is an important factor, as we shall see.

Now, if a zero begins to appear with unusual consistency in your life, then the Cosmos is trying to tell you something. This number may be your Angel Number. Like all Angel Numbers, it may not appear by itself but as part of numbers that keep showing up, such as a house number, a phone number with several zeros, or a car number with a zero in it. There are several ways in which this might occur. If you are aware of the value of numbers, then you are sure to spot its recurrence.

Zeros' appearing likely means to continue doing what you're doing. It emphasizes this; go ahead with complete confidence. Your Angel Guides are with you. It is time to check your options and make the right decision. Be sure that the Angels are on your side and are guiding you. Just follow their lead. Any difficulties which you might be up against are going to go away.

Number 1, if it manifests, means a spiritual change is in the air.

If you keep waking up at night and see that the hour is 11 or that minute hand indicates 11 minutes, that is a sign that the Cosmos is trying to send a message. It could be your Angel Number. If so, it is important to pay attention to it and what it is trying to say. It is likely telling you that a change is coming, and you need to prepare for it. Trust and remain positive. Your Angel Guides are there to help your progress on your path!

Let us now consider Number 2.

If twos appear regularly, it indicates the spirit world is telling you to go ahead and make your dream world a reality. This is a time to reflect and work towards goals. It must be noted that the sum of two 2s makes four, which has links to hard work and due diligence. The appearance of '2' often means that new relationships are about to form. The perspectives of others need to be heeded at this time.

The Number 3 as the Angel Number.

This number suggests that you are in spiritual alignment. The three vibrations mean the time is ripe to pursue your purpose in life, don't hold back your self-expression. It is also an indication to try and connect with the Higher Masters.

The Number 4 as the Angel Number.

The appearance of '4' means that you are being loved by your Angel Guide. The difficulties you may be going through are temporary. Your spirit guide will provide the energy and power to get through them successfully. Be reassured. Try and meditate so that your mind focuses on higher energies.

The Number 5 as the Angel Number.

When this number seems like your Angel Number, then take it as a symbol of good tidings. It is essentially a sign that you must pause and examine your path. It tells you to be aware that new things are about to happen. Make sure that your diet is healthy and nutritious. Health is one of the areas where caution is indicated when a plethora of '5's appears. However, it means that positive changes are coming. Just be physically and mentally ready for them.

The Number 6 as the Angel Number.

This sign means the time has come to heal yourself; essentially, heal the Soul. This really means letting the light of the spirit within, which is the Soul, shine forth. Remove the grossness of life which covers it. Difficult times you are probably going through need some inner light to show the way. This is a time to focus on balance.

The Number 7 as the Angel Number.

This number means that the Angels have blessed you. They are looking out for you and helping changes happen. Mainly, these are spiritual changes. To be prepared for these changes and deal with them successfully, it is time to engage in spiritual activities such as prayer and meditation. It may also be a good idea to study spiritual books. Keep your heart and your mind open to vibrations from the Cosmos. They are coming, and you, as the recipient, must be ready. A good idea would be to do yoga exercises and realign, especially those which enhance concentration and focus.

The Number 8 as the Angel Number.

Initially, this indicates periods of difficulty and strain, but perseverance with whatever you do helps overcome the issues. This number shows that hard work and determination can conquer most hurdles. It is important to keep in mind that the Angel Guides are watching, and they will assist you in your work towards success. However, you must be careful not to be too involved in material gains; otherwise, trouble lies ahead. You are not in sync with the Universe. Practice moderation at all times, be discerning and careful.

The Number 9 as the Angel Number.

When this number appears in your life, be ready for a profound spiritual awakening and change in your life pattern. The number nine is a magic number and a highly potent symbol of spirituality. It is, in fact, the magic number of alchemy. It is the triplicity of the original Trinity, hence its power and importance. The Cosmic Powers seem to be pointing at a shift from the ordinary, material life to a higher plane of existence. The inner-light or spirit which resides in you is about to shine forth in all its glory. Give it the chance to do so - practice compassion. Work on your inward journeys as much as possible. Meditation is the best way to do this. You will perceive that the feelings and visions during meditation undergo a sea of change. Take note of what exactly is happening, and the answer will come to you.

To conclude, it is necessary to point out that the Angel Number indications provided are a starting point or a guideline that can be used to decode the meaning of the number which begins to appear uncannily in your life. It is necessary to interpret them to fit your life's issues. This can be achieved through meditation, and as mentioned earlier, through a keen awareness of your surroundings. Close contact with Nature is an excellent way to develop this connection with Divine Energy. That's the source of the numbers. The retraction of the conscious mind for periods of time is required to feel the presence of the spirit. Keep in mind that the number you believe is your Angel Number must be recurring. Just a one-off sighting may not mean anything at all. The best way is to seek seclusion once in a while. Solitude is excellent for spiritual gains. The constant noise, part of our modern-day life, is a distraction. Switch off cell phones for several hours. This is your private time. No intrusions are allowed.

Sometimes, mixed numbers appear to manifest themselves. This needs a different type of interpretation. Each number, especially the Core Number, needs to be identified and understood.

The appearance of Angel Numbers may at times disappear. You may think that the Divine has abandoned you. That is not the case. There are reasons why Angel Numbers sometimes leave you. Some of the important reasons include:

- Negative thoughts and speech.

- Sense of overpowering frustration.
- Feeling of fear arising out of adverse circumstances.
- Bouts of anger.

Life does not always go according to plan. Situations arise out of nowhere and can throw everything out of kilt. This is normal, and it has to be dealt with. That's the way life works. Therefore, if your Angel Number has done a disappearing act, stay calm, practice meditation, say your prayers asking for guidance, and it is sure to return. It does not mean that your spiritual awakening process is going awry. It is just possible that your Angel Number is about to change to reflect your changing spiritual attainments. Have patience and watch for new numbers. They are sure to appear! It is also possible that your old Angel Number reappears. The main idea is not to worry or become stressed; that's a negative way of handling things. In the spiritual world, not everything moves linearly. Life, too, is sometimes not linear. The new theory, called the "Chaos Theory," says just that.

Something minimal might lead to more significant ramifications. The small things generally escape our attention. Only when the bigger event happens do we realize where it all started. The spiritual journey is one where pauses in progress happen. This is not a sign that something has gone wrong; it is simply how it works. It is necessary to keep that in mind at all times. The awakening process may be now getting ready to move to another plane, a higher one. Silence of the spirit precedes such an event.

Dealing With Complex Numbers: (From the Author's book, "Spiritual Meaning of Numbers")

When you are faced with complex numbers, such as 924 or something similar, the **First Step** is to figure out the meanings indicated by each individual number.

'Nine' energies are forgiveness, compassion, community, reward, and lethargy.

The energies of 'two' are summed up by sensitivity, compromise, harmony, and balance.

'Four' energies are summed up by stability, tradition, hard work, security, and unchangeability.

Second Step:

- Take note of the arrangement of these three numbers.
- Note that 'nine' may be the potential number identifying the context or cause of this Angel Number.
- Think about how the energies of 'two' may be defining the main drive or point of the Angel Number. The 'four' may be the results of 'nine' and 'two', or it could be an explanation of how the number 'two' influences your life.

'Nine' as the Causal Number: You are emerging from the end of one cycle and are entering another.

'Two' as Core Number: You are loved and supported by the Universe, spirit guides, deceased loved ones, and your earthly community.

'Four' as an Effect Number: Get down to work. Use skills and organization to achieve your dreams.

Third Step: Research and consider the additional meanings of other number combinations within your Angel Number. They may point you in different directions.

92: You are moving from a stage of spiritual completion and are being encouraged to continue pursuing spiritual harmony and balance.

24: As you focus on your work (both spiritual and physical), your Angel Guides support you.

Fourth Step: Calculate the cumulative (or hidden) number of your Angel Number by adding all of the numbers together and then adding the sum as well. However, if the cumulative sum is '11', '22', or '33', don't continue with the calculation since these numbers are significant and powerful.

(924 = 9+2+4 = 15* = 1 + 5 = 6)

As stated previously, if the number '15' were '11', '22', or '33', many numerologists would recommend stopping your calculations, as these are master numbers, but it really is up to you! In this calculation, our cumulative (or hidden) Core Number is 'six,' which relates to balancing and reassessing one's priorities.

Fifth Step: Meditate and analyze the various meanings and applications found in all of these numbers. Synthesize what you have discovered into intentional messages of positivity and manifestation.

A potential reading for '924' could be: As you emerge from the end of one cycle and enter another one, know that you are loved and supported by your angels. With this knowledge, embrace empowerment and healthy balance within life as you continue working on your path to manifestation and success.

You could turn this into intentional speech for manifestation techniques is to add 'I' to these statements and personalize the expression of the numbers' energies. For example: "I am loved! I am ready for a new phase of life! I embrace power and balance as I manifest my dreams!"

Be flexible enough to interpret these numbers to fit your present state. It reflects your current position and offers a way out. Put the two together, and you have your answer.

Chapter 7
Letting Go

The question here is, what does "letting go" really mean? Well, it's one of the most essential ideas for attaining peace and harmony in your life.

Ask a person what they want the most, and chances are they will say 'peace.' Some, of course, will say 'happiness.' The path to either of these desired states consists of:

- Changing fixed ideas and thoughts in the conscious mind.
- Reducing craving and attachment towards external objects.
- Becoming good with or without.

Let us see how the mind can be changed so that embedded concepts can be modified to allow for more of the forces of peace and happiness to enter.

Now the first thing is to know that no matter who you are, you have specific fixed ideas in your head which more or less color all your decisions and perceptions. These are part of the conscious mind and are active all the time. Previous thoughts, events, and ideas are built into the conscious mind. When something new happens, the conscious mind uses this template to analyze the event, whatever it may be. This means that a fixed set of ideas is running your vision in life.

When something goes wrong, depending on how you handled a similar situation before, the conscious mind might throw up a response such as, 'I knew I wasn't up to it,' or something similar. This is your built-in response acting. It is time to get rid of some of these damaging mindsets. They morph and distort your worldview.

This can be achieved by asking yourself questions. Now, the conscious mind will always respond in the same way. It is to the unconscious mind that you must now turn. There lies the truth of the matter. The best way is to sit quietly and meditate. Ask yourself how you can react differently. Wait for the answer. The unconscious will respond, but it needs time. It has to get past the conscious mind to get this answer through to you. Then there is the ego. The ego wants to retain its position as the primary influencer of decisions. It won't let go easily, either.

Let's say you often think that 'I don't have enough. Now the word 'enough' is a tricky one. When you say, "I do not have enough," do you mean not enough when compared to so-and-so or such and such? Normally, this is the case. But, a hungry man, when he says, "I don't have enough," means something completely different.

Now, comparisons with people who have more than you have is a disastrous mental position. It is never satisfying. Ask yourself whether you really need additional stuff to make you happy. Let's work through this idea a little more.

You buy that fancy Italian sofa set you think you should have to rival something similar that you saw at a friend's house. You set up the sofa, and you think you feel happy? Why? Because now when your guests come, they will praise your taste in furniture. It is the praise that makes you feel good. But, after several visits, that praise will disappear. Will you still be happy? Remember, no more praise. The answer is 'no.' That object has lost its glory or numinosity. The thought process that made you buy the sofa needs to change, but the rationale behind the decision must be destroyed.

Consider this: the old sofa which you replaced with the fancy Italian job; was it damaged or, in any way, degraded so that it was unserviceable? No? Then the decision to replace it was just to garner some words of praise? Does that sound very clever or rational? In plain terms, it sounds silly. Once you understand this, the idea of competing with people will slowly go away. That is what is meant by reorganizing your thoughts. You get rid of the cobwebs in your mind which clutter up your life.

There are many similar ideas which are there. They need to be examined and removed, or at best, modified. Your entire life perspective needs to undergo a change, retaining only that which is good.

This process of reorienting your mind is an essential step towards spiritual awakening. It is a process that must be undertaken simultaneously. Typically, everyone's mind is filled with the trivial debris of everyday life, along with inhibitions and other complexities. Cleansing the mind of all unnecessary and detrimental thoughts is a must. However, be aware that removing some complexities is not easy. It takes time and real effort, but it can be done.

Once the cleansing process begins, the body starts to feel lighter, and the mind also seems to be happier. This is because these thoughts and ideas were weighing down on the mind and the body.

The human mind is subject to several emotions. These can seriously affect our lives and not always for the better.

Let's start with the feeling of fear, a primal emotion, and which everyone has. It is almost certain that everyone has a fear of something. Sometimes the fear is there but not easily recognized. That does not mean it does not exist. But fears which are consciously present need to be dealt with. One of the ways is to face it head-on. Stand up to it and ask why? What is it that scares you? If you do this whenever the fear appears, the chances are that the problem will resolve itself. Usually, these are psychological projections. Once identified, they can be handled and removed. Fear of the unknown is the most common fear which people have. C. G. Jung gave this fear a name: 'misoneism.'

An excellent way to understand the basis and nature of your fears is to sit down and write them. Describe them in detail and see what happens. Sometimes, the very act of writing things down reveals the real nature of it. It is quite possible that the fear may turn out to be something trivial. Once this recognition takes place, the fear disappears.

However, it is possible that while writing about a particular fear, some other fear begins to emerge. It is something that was there but not recognized. Sort of like in the back of the mind, that fear arose from the unconscious. The only way to deal with this kind of fear is to let it surface into the conscious mind and then deal with it. Meditation is a great help in resolving these fears. Meditation brings these fears up to the conscious mind, and over time, they play out and just go away. They lose their psychic energy.

Understanding why a particular fear exists is also an effective tool. For example, you have always been afraid before a test or an examination of any kind. Ask yourself if the fear was justified. Think back to the results. Were they bad? If not, then the fear is irrational. Get rid of it by telling yourself that you were fooled into being scared. There is nothing like self-teasing to get rid of unnecessary things.

A good way of tackling fears is to force yourself to stay calm and open to positive influences. Look at the flowers or play some soothing music. Not all fears go away quickly. Some are deep-rooted and take time to eradicate, but you need to make an effort to remove them continuously. Never let the appearance of a fear go unchallenged.

If these dark episodes threaten to take over your life, concentrate on the spiritual awakening side of things. Meditate and pray. Both are capable of miracles. Depend upon it. Also, try and engage in helping others, reaching out to people who need your assistance. These positive energies need to be multiplied so that the negative energies become less powerful to cause trouble. Fear is negative energy. It has to be overcome.

As mentioned earlier, meditation brings to the surface these dark fears. However, once you let them play themselves out, you are rid of them.

Fill your life with love. This can be love for your family, friends and love for all of Creation. Your whole perception of life will undergo a radical transformation. These are positive energies; cultivate them!

Grief is a compelling emotion and can cast a long shadow on your life. It is essential to get past it and move on. Let's see some of the ways you can do this.

When an event causes grief, and it is most often the passing away of someone close which brings it on, grieve without hesitation. Let it all pour out. Cry as much as you want. It is the outpouring that will later help to reduce the pain. However, keeping it in is dangerous. It tends to stay for a long time, if not forever.

It is said that time is the great healer and that the passage of time heals all. While this is mostly true, it isn't always the case. Sometimes, the intense grief sinks into the unconscious and stays there, occasionally surfacing to cause extreme pain. However, it generally appears when least expected. For example, a strain of music or a particular smell can trigger the emotion. Therefore, it is necessary to deal with it as quickly as possible.

The first step in dealing with grief is to understand that what happened has happened. The departed soul has left this plane, but they are forever with you in spirit. It is the journey of life. That being said, life for the survivors must go on. No matter who they were, the departed soul would certainly not want you to ruin your life. They would like you to carry on regardless. So it would be best if you moved forward. Remind yourself whenever you feel a sense of grief surfacing that they may be gone in body but are forever with you in spirit. Let it out, take a deep breath and carry on, as they would want you to.

Making some changes in your life could help. When people close to you pass away, they leave a vacuum that needs filling. Since nature abhors vacuums, it will tend to drag you into that void, so fill it by changing small things in your life. One of the ways this can be done is to take up a new hobby and reset your goals in life. Work towards new ideas and priorities. The spiritual awakening you are undergoing is an excellent help in realigning your mind.

From the mind and its concepts and emotions, we move on to letting go of material objects.

Letting go does not mean throwing away. It means being less in love with the things, less attached. Life without material objects would be impossible, at least life as it is today. Everyone needs a place to stay, some furniture in the home, and possibly a car or a bicycle to move around - the basics.

So, then, what is "letting go"? Letting go means to mentally consider these objects as just objects and not something you absolutely must hang on to. A strong attachment to material objects means that the veil of illusion still controls the mind. You need to remove this intense feeling of attachment. They don't really belong to you; you are just the caretaker, here for a short time. When you depart, you cannot take anything with you. If you can't take it with you, it never was yours. Get rid of that illusion. It tends to take your vision away from far more important and beautiful ideas and feelings. Once the sense of "letting go" starts, life becomes much calmer and more peaceful. It is as if a weight has just rolled off your shoulders. It is a noticeable feeling. After the first step, the rest comes automatically. You cannot afford this weight if you aim to connect with the higher powers spiritually.

Along with attachment, let go of control. Like the illusion of possession, control, too, is an illusion. You may feel that you have control over this and that. You don't. Things tend to work better when control is absent. That means your control. If the process is correct, the results will appear. If you have a tendency to control, this means that you are afraid of the outcome. This is a feeling of fear. This fear makes a person a controlling type; another aspect is power. Control over anything is a feeling of power. It is a feeling that wants to master the outcome of everything in a specific manner that is satisfactory to the controller. But as we all know, nothing in this world is sure. Things have an inherent tendency to go awry, as they do. That's a fact of life. The problem is that controlling people are challenging to deal with. They have closed minds and live in their own fantasy world.

Letting go of control releases tensions in the mind and body. It is incredibly beneficial to surrender and see what happens. It actually gives better results than control. Nature sometimes rewards those in tune with Her and do not want to bend Her to their will.

Surrender means non-action. The question to ask yourself is why you want to have control. It could be the anxiety that something may go wrong or just a pathological need. Control is generally backed by strong emotion, either fear or power. In case it is fear, that is easy to handle. However, if it is pathological, then it is far more complicated. It is a good idea to be watchful but not controlling. Being watchful usually works just as well.

Giving up control is initially difficult. It is an ingrained habit, and habits die hard, as we all know. But it can be done. Start with a small thing. Let go, and see what happens. Did everything go haywire? No? Then why bother to control and bring on stress? Control does bring on enormous pressure as the mind grapples with the uncertainty of the outcome. You really don't need this, and as you will gradually realize, giving up control does not mean devastation! It just means a more relaxed and stress-free life. Controlling parents face rebellion from their children sooner or later; the stress gets to them, too!

That's the problem with control. It affects the controller as well as the person being controlled. So let's do without it. Set your mind free, and enjoy the feeling of lightness and peace.

An ancient savant once said, "Worldly people lose their roots, and cling onto the treetops." Remember this whenever you want to exercise control and get too heavily involved in the material world.

Let us now look at some practices that are part of a spiritual awakening. There are mentions of these in the earlier chapters, but we just focus on the practical aspects here.

Step One: Sit down and think. Are you ready for this? Keep the book by your side if you need to refresh your mind about what you are doing. If you feel resolute enough, great! Time to start.

Step Two: Sit in solitude. Ideally, find a place in your house which you can use regularly. Sit down and relax. Switch off your mobile phone - or put it on silent - and put it where you can't see it. Your mind must be free of distractions. Now think about the spiritual awakening process. Most of the time, the conscious mind, which wants to be involved with external phenomena, will try to make you feel bored. Your mind may say, "What the heck are you doing sitting here?". Tell yourself that this is a journey you are determined to make. Once your mind accepts that it cannot divert you from the course, you are ready to start.

Sitting in complete solitude is the way forward - always. Initially, sitting in solitude is the training that you must practice. The conscious mind needs to be subdued during this period. Silence is the main thing here. Silence, as opposed to continuous noise, is the necessary ingredient. Think of music; if it were not for the spaces of silence between notes, the whole thing would just be a cacophony of noise that would drive anyone crazy after a few seconds. That's why periods of silence are required. These periods do an important thing: they make your life's vibrations more stable.

Once you can sit in solitude, start the process of meditation. In the beginning, this essentially means sitting peacefully in one place without interruption. It is advisable to sit on the floor; however, a chair may be used. Try not to think of anything in particular. Notice the images that are whizzing through your mind. Let them go. They need to play themselves out. The idea that you must come to a point where your mind is blank is nonsense. The whole idea is to allow the images and thoughts from the conscious and the unconscious mind to reduce their energy levels. So just let them go. After a few days, you will find that these images are slowing down. They are losing their psychic energy.

Once the images have slowed down, try to think of some image, whether of God, a saint you revere, or just a beautiful aspect of Mother Nature. **Hold this image and meditate on it.** Do not try to analyze anything. Just hold the image in your mind as long as you can. Your unconscious mind will slowly use these periods of meditation to tell you many things. Not verbally, of course, the unconscious does not speak; it sends its messages as psychic feelings. There is an important point here. Try to use the same place every day, and the meditation practice must be regular to get its benefits. Irregular meditation does not work. The chain is broken.

Along with meditation, practice a few other practical things like helping others, the needy, and those who require assistance. Bring joy into the lives of others and watch that joy spill over into you. It works like magic. This upliftment of mood helps in spiritual progress. The cobwebs of worry and stress, the visible aspects of life, need to be reduced. They are the things blocking the inner light, the Pure Spirit, and connection, which is the sole aim of a spiritual awakening.

Go on a trip and stay amidst Nature for some time. The place where you go must be free from crowds. You need solitude to commune with Mother Nature. If you can, meditate. The benefits are enormous. The Spirit within you is abundantly present in Mother Nature. Try and connect with it, and let your intuition guide you. The unconscious will activate your intuitive faculty.

Most people feel a strange power when alone with Nature, deep inside a forest, or in the mountains. Any mountaineer knows and feels the power of some invisible spirit, which seems to permeate the place. Some even pay obeisance to the Spirit. The local people are conversant with this presence and never move without praying to it. Living with nature gives these locals a sense of the Divine. In some cultures, people offer a prayer to the Sea God before entering the sea, whether to swim or fish. The Great Spirit rules everything it feels. The Native Americans knew this and prayed and offered tobacco so that the Spirit would keep them safe.

The trick is to work at it quietly and patiently. It takes time, but the rewards are worth it. If you have dark thoughts in the initial periods of meditation, don't worry. It's natural, and you need to get rid of the baggage. They will vanish over time, but you just need to hold steadfast to your target.

Simplify life's needs. You may be surprised by how little you actually need. You will feel the lightness of a simple life. Your shoulders will feel less heavy. Try it!

What has been said so far is a guide. It is the way to see where the path to spiritual awakening might lie. However, the journey must be yours and only yours. Use the tools wisely and with conviction, and changes will happen. Remember that these changes are spiritual and do not follow a timetable. They just happen at their own pace. So, do not be disheartened at slow progress. Slow does not mean failure.

The secret is to live every moment, savor every moment. That's the core teaching of the Japanese philosophy called 'Bushido.' So follow it as much as you can.

Conclusion

If you have come this far, you are aware of what a spiritual awakening is all about and what you need to do. You have read about the techniques which are to be used and the results of those practices.

Remember that what you are doing is an ancient technique; it is something with a pedigree. The process of looking inward has been practiced for centuries, so it is a proven way to attain an elevated frame of mind and a more peaceful and cognizant way of life. This book just puts it all together for you.

Now you understand the importance of numbers and the various signs and symbols that the Cosmic Forces send. These are important, and once you have started on your spiritual journey, use these hints from the Divine to guide you.

Make sure that the sightings are meant for you, and see if they tend to repeat. If they are messages, they have a tendency to repeat themselves. As your awareness grows through the medium of meditation, you will know which is a sign meant for you and which is not.

The important thing to remember is this: use the data provided for each symbol, number, animal, bird, and insect as a hint. First, however, try and see how it applies to you. These symbols generally signify ideas meant for you alone. The unconscious mind will take some time to tell you what it means. If necessary, keep a journal of what you saw and when.

Remember that the conscious mind will try its best to interpret the signs and symbols that you begin to notice. Just keep it in mind and go about your work. When you sit down to meditate, try and think of the sign. Try and visualize it.

It may take a couple of meditation sessions to get the answer, but be patient; it will come. First, it needs to slowly send messages to the conscious mind, which you will then know. The unconscious is a very deep area of the mind. It has many critical secret matters which you will slowly get to know as your spiritual awakening progresses.

The other important thing is being aware that you are in the process of tapping into the unconscious part of your mind. This part of the mind, though unknown, is extremely potent. If specific terrifying memories surface, as indicated in the text, ignore them. This means just to let them float across. They will slowly go away. This is just a reminder.

Read your entries in the journal once a day, at least. It is a good idea to read it just before you sit for meditation. It's a renewal of data that the unconscious mind will use. Just keep in mind that the results may not be instantaneous - the unconscious works in mysterious ways. The trick is to let it.

It is also crucial to track your dreams. Visions of symbols, such as those mentioned in this book, also have significance. Enter the content of the dreams in the journal, too. There will come a moment, when you least expect it, that you will know their significance. Wait for that flash of illumination. You cannot control it, be patient. It will appear sooner or later.

Try and simplify your life as much as possible. A simple life is less of a burden to bear, and you want to eliminate all the unnecessary stresses.

There are many other ideas in this book about awakening your inner self. That's what this text is all about.

Just bear in mind that this is an inward journey. It is a journey that will connect you to your inner self, the Pure Spirit. Once you connect even briefly to this inner light, your life will change for the better. You will enjoy a different and new kind of peace and happiness of a more permanent kind. So work towards your goal with concentration and patience. You are sure to reach it.

A spiritual awakening is something that will make your life more beautiful, and more importantly, complete. The unconscious is necessary in one's life. Once the unconscious begins to function, new vistas will open up, and life, in general, will start to appear to be something grand. The drama of life will have a new meaning.

The fact that you want a spiritual awakening means that something inside you is talking to you. Your time has come, as the mystics say, to make the change. So, follow that voice. It is the Divine speaking to you. Have no doubt whatsoever about that.

The book you are holding has a detailed account of how to achieve this. It mentions the required systems, the signs and symbols that become relevant, and some of the issues that must be overcome. Follow the guidelines, and you will undoubtedly see success. Your feelings will tell you that you have made it.

A Free Gift for You!

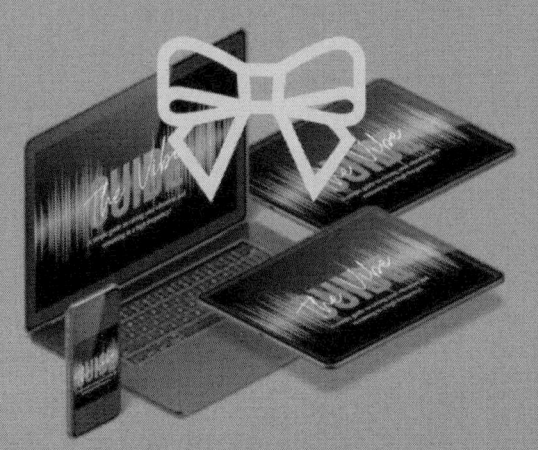

In the "**Vibe Guide**," you will learn...

- 15 techniques to raise your vibrations and stay in a high frequency
- How to manifest your desires
- How to find peace...

and so much more!

Go to bellemotley.com to receive your free gift!

www.bellemotley.com

References

Browning, R. *Paracelsus*. London, Methuen & Co, 1909.

Freud, S. et al. *The Major Works of Sigmund Freud*. Chicago, William Benton, 1952.

Jung, C. G., & Violet S. *The Basic Writings of C.G. Jung*. New York, Modern Library, 1959.

P Lal. *The Bhagavad Gita*. Delhi, Roli; Lancaster, 2005.

Pseud. Sepharial. *The Kabala of Numbers... A Handbook of Interpretation ... New Edition, Enlarged and Revised*. Pt. 1. Pp. 204. William Rider & Son: London, 1914.

Raynor, Carey J. *The Imprisoned Splendour: An Approach to Reality, Based upon the Significance of Data Drawn from the Fields of Natural Science, Psychical Research and Mystical Experience*. London, Hodder and Stoughton, 1953.

Rocke, A. J., and Inc Ebrary. *Image and Reality : Kekulé, Kopp, and the Scientific Imagination*. Chicago; London, The University Of Chicago Press, 2010.

Ryan, R. E. *The Great Circle: Shamanism and the Psychology of C.G. Jung*. London, Vega, 2002.

"Spiritual Meaning of Seeing a Feather - Meaning of Black, Blue, Purple & Different Color Feathers." *California Psychics*, 19 Nov. 2020, www.californiapsychics.com/blog/animal-sightings-symbolism/meaning-feather-sighting.html.

Watts, Alan. *The Book on the Taboo against Knowing Who You Are*. London, Souvenir Press, 2012.

"THE FEYNMAN SERIES - Curiosity." *Www.youtube.com*, 2 Oct. 2011, www.youtube.com/watch?v=lmTmGLzPVyM. Accessed 7 Dec. 2021.

Motley, B. (2021). *The Spiritual Meanings of Numbers*. Spiritual Growth.

Made in the USA
Columbia, SC
23 February 2022